Your simple
Healthy Teeth and Heal
Without Tre

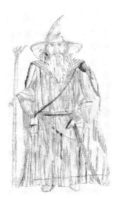

Something To Chew On

A new and holistic mind/body approach to dental health and general health based on simplicity and personal power

Easy to Understand and Easy to Master

By

Philip Christie
B.A., B.Dent.Sc., M.A., M.Dent.Sc.

© Copyright 2003 Philip Christie. All rights reserved.

No part of this publication may be reproduced, stored in a retrieval system, or transmitted, in any form or by any means, electronic, mechanical, photocopying, recording, or otherwise, without the written prior permission of the author.

Printed in Victoria, Canada

Note for Librarians: a cataloguing record for this book that includes Dewey Classification and US Library of Congress numbers is available from the National Library of Canada. The complete cataloguing record can be obtained from the National Library's online database at:
www.nlc-bnc.ca/amicus/index-e.html
ISBN 1-4120-1381-x

TRAFFORD

This book was published on-demand in cooperation with Trafford Publishing.
On-demand publishing is a unique process and service of making a book available for retail sale to the public taking advantage of on-demand manufacturing and Internet marketing. On-demand publishing includes promotions, retail sales, manufacturing, order fulfilment, accounting and collecting royalties on behalf of the author.

Suite 6E, 2333 Government St., Victoria, B.C. V8T 4P4, CANADA
Phone   250-383-6864   Toll-free 1-888-232-4444 (Canada & US)
Fax 250-383-6804   E-mail sales@trafford.com   Web site
www.trafford.com
TRAFFORD PUBLISHING IS A DIVISION OF TRAFFORD HOLDINGS LTD.
Trafford Catalogue #03-1759   www.trafford.com/robots/03-1759.html

10   9   8   7   6   5   4

Lovingly dedicated to the spirits of my father Pilib, and my sisters Sharon and Nóirín.

About The Author

Philip Christie is a native of Finglas, North Dublin and was educated at St. Vincent's C.B.S., Glasnevin. He was conferred with a Bachelor's Degree in Dental Science at Trinity College Dublin in 1980. His research in the field of Periodontology earned him a Masters Degree in Dental Science, again from Trinity College Dublin in 1995. His main interest in dental health has always been in the prevention of disease.

Currently based in Waterford City, Philip Christie brings to the practice of Dentistry a holistic and people-centered approach. Through his easy and friendly manner and deep understanding of the issues that lie behind dental disease, he helps dissolve the fears and phobias which traditionally surround a dental visit. The insights shared in this work form the basis for the Integrated Model of Dental Care which this author brings to the field of Dental Science.

Acknowledgements

With grateful thanks to my family who supported and helped me every step of the way. Thanks to Mag, my partner, who always gives 100% commitment to our projects. Thanks to Maggie for constructive criticism as well as her encouragement and support. Thanks to Philip for the title (so apt) and his belief in me. Thanks to James, our youngest, who proved the power of personal choice in action by becoming a great little artist at age 9 and supplying the drawings. I have included these drawings because they are testament to the innate ability of the human being to succeed by willingness, courage, determination and commitment. James actually believed that he could not draw!!

Thanks to my mother, sisters and brother for their support and encouragement. Thanks to my mother-in-law Breda Howe for her constant support and for finding Trafford Publishing for us. Thanks to Mag for proof-reading and suggestions. Thanks to my sister, Deirdre for her proof-reading and editing contribution (an excellent job!). Thanks also to my good friend John for his help in revising and corrections.

A special thank you to Ray and Patricia Bassett for their long, close and enduring friendship.

Thanks as well to my dear friends Peadar and Terry Clarke, always available for advice, and all my friends connected with the Lourdes Kindness Pilgrimage. Thanks to all my many dear friends for their love and support. In all, I have been truly blessed.

I would like to express my deep gratitude to my many teachers, friends and colleagues at the School of Dental Science, Trinity College Dublin and the Dublin Dental Hospital. I feel particularly grateful to Professor Liam McDevitt and Professor Noel Claffey for their kindness to me as well as their excellent teaching from their vast resources of knowledge and experience.

My grateful thanks are due, in a very special way, to the courage and commitment of other wonderful teachers/authors who have dared to speak of new ways of thinking and being. These pioneers renewed my hope and fostered in me, my own inner desire to see beyond the "obvious" and bring solutions to seemingly intractable problems.

Thanks to Deepak Chopra, M.D., Caroline Myss, PhD., Larry Dossey, M.D., Anthony Robbins, Ken Carey, Patrick Francis, Colin Tipping, Joan Borysenko, PhD., Ryuho Okawa, Neale Donald Walshe, Sogyal Rinpoche, Mikhael Aivanhov, Helen Schucman and Bill Thetford, Thich Nhat Hanh, Jon Kabat-Zinn, Barbara Ann Brennan and Saundra Stephen.

Grateful thanks to Professor Herbert Benson and his "Wellness Team" at Harvard Medical School and in particular to Annie Webster, PhD. and the Cardiac Wellness team with whom I was fortunate enough to have direct tuition. Professor Benson and his team have produced a comprehensive medical model of Wellness and Health Promotion, which has the potential to reform any ailing Health Service to the benefit of both the healthcare professionals and the people they serve.

All drawings courtesy of James Christie, aged nine years.

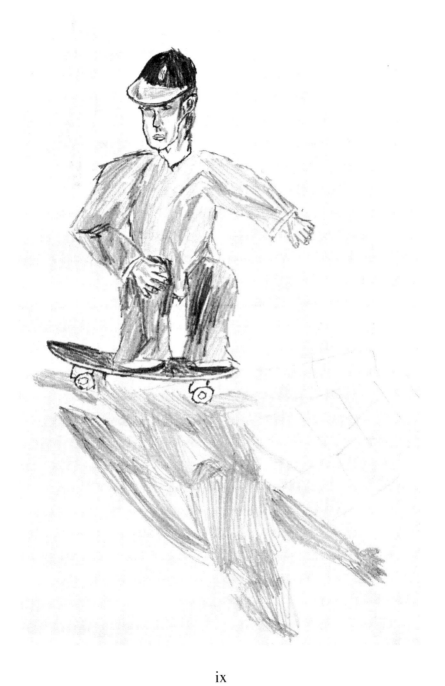

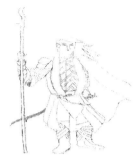

Table of Contents

About the Author   Page   v

Acknowledgements   Page   vii

A Teacher's Comment   Page   xiii

Foreword   Page   xv

Introduction To The Concept   Page   xvii

How to Use the Manual   Page   xxi

Chapter 1.
    Do You Mind?   Page   1

Chapter 2.
    Feelings - Nothing More Than Feelings?   Page   9

Chapter 3.
    To Do or Not to Do?   Page   17

Chapter 4.
    Speak Your Mind!   Page   27

Chapter 5.
    Other Habits Affecting The Teeth   Page 35

Chapter 6.
    Putting It All Together   Page 43

Chapter 7.
    Where Do I Begin   Page 49

Chapter 8.
    Preventing Tooth Decay   Page 61

Chapter 9.
    Preventing Gum Disease   Page 69

Chapter 10.
    Joint And Muscle Problems   Page 83

Chapter 11.
    Toothbrush Damage   Page 89

Chapter 12.
    Acid Damage   Page 95

Chapter 13.
    Prevention For Children   Page 101

Chapter 14.
    The Mouth is the Mirror   Page 113

Chapter 15.
    What's It All About, Anyway?   Page 123

A Teacher's Comment

As a teacher having read Dr. Christie's book I was struck by its gentleness and simplicity in dealing with what could be a highly complex subject matter. After 25 years in a classroom and being aware of the physical and emotional backgrounds of the children, I have seen first hand evidence of what Dr. Christie describes in his book. One need only take a look at the contents of the lunch-boxes in a classroom on any given day. I recommend this book without reservation to all parents and teachers and suggest that this would be an excellent reference book for any Social, Personal and Health Education programme (S.P.H.E.)

John Walshe, Primary Teacher

Foreword

The healthcare systems of all first world countries have much in common. They are all in crisis. They use a model that is based on medical hierarchy and multi-layered administration. There is no sign of a solution. If anything, we can expect worse. All this has been predicted for the past twenty years or more. Compelling reasons were given and possible solutions were offered. It hardly mattered. Nobody listened. Now we profess that we are surprised, even puzzled, at the demise of the great dreams - that science would conquer illness and that high quality health-care would be easily accessible by everyone.

It could be different. Many far-seeing individuals have pointed out that medicine must first of all be patient- based. That is hardly asking a lot. But what does it mean to be patient-focused? It requires that we embrace the *totality* of each individual - body mind and spirit. While it is desirable to observe the best principles of science, we must use them appropriately and responsibly. That in turn means allowing medical technology, whether machinery, procedures or medicines, a rightful but confined role in medical care. In acute illness, these technologies can be life saving and produce outcomes bordering on the miraculous. Yet we have allowed ourselves to be seduced by their power. Thus we end up treating all forms of illness with the same methodology, an approach that is often inappropriate and always expensive. We have somehow lost our way.

Science has very little to say about the mind, particularly the emotions - and nothing at all to say concerning spirit. This need not be a problem. Scientific method stands on its own. It underpins much of what is good about modern medicine. Yet it does not take sides. It is about accuracy and truth. Medical Scientific Dogma, on the other hand, is willing to pronounce on everything it encounters. What it cannot measure it considers unimportant. By inference then, a large portion of what makes us full human beings is not worthy of so-called scientific study or comment. This thinking dominates health systems, both in the practice of medicine and the delivery of care. There is no room for partnership with the patient in this model. He/she is peripheral. It is prohibitively expensive too, using valuable technology to treat the *effects*, when it should be looking at the *causes* of illness.

Integrated medical models offer a different approach. The patient is involved fully in the management of the illness on the one hand and in the active promotion of health on the other. There is a recognition of the innate ability of each person to participate in the healing process. Through a variety of techniques that are easily taught, the patient is *empowered.* This book describes such an approach. In language that is easily understood, Dr. Philip Christie outlines some of these methods and how to use them. We need books like this.

Dr. Paddy Rudden, General Medical Practitioner

Introduction To The Concept

This manual is for you, the individual person.

The purpose of the manual is to give you what rightfully belongs to you - the Captaincy of your own ship. The dentist may help you along the way but you are the "boss". You are the Captain of your Ship.

The Captain makes the decisions. He/she listens carefully to the advice of others but the decision or choice is always a matter finally for the Captain.

Your biggest and best resource is yourself. The manual is intended as practical and everyday. It is easy to implement. It costs little to implement. All that is required of you is care, willingness, commitment, and time.

The approach that we will offer is quite different from the usual approaches to dental disease. Traditionally the focus is on the teeth and what can be done to them. The dentist finds the problems and then fixes them. The person has the minor role while the dentist has the major one. This model serves to keep the focus on the dentist and away from the person and so tends to promote dependence rather than independence.

Holistic Dentistry - Understanding The Whole Person.

We offer a new way, one where the person assumes the major role and the dentist the minor one. We offer a mind/body or holistic approach. It views the person as a whole, mind and body. It allows us to look anew and reinterpret the well-known characteristics of dental disease through understanding a little more of our basic human nature.

Although much has been spoken and written of mind/body approaches I am not aware of a clear documentation of pathways between mind and body. I hope to show such a clear pathway. Many have had difficulty understanding how mind, which is so non-physical, could be related to the physical body. Indeed mind has readily been put down as 'not real'. How often have you heard people say " that is **only** in your **mind**" clearly implying "that is **not real**".

I will point a clear pathway of **cause** and **effect**.

We begin with the mind, - our thoughts, ideas, notions and attitudes about ourselves. In particular it is the *__negative__* **thoughts, ideas, notions** and **attitudes** that do not serve either our general good or our good health.

We will then follow these negative thoughts, ideas, notions etc. and see how they can influence our **feelings** and **emotions** negatively. Then we will see how our **emotional well-being** relates to what is called **stress**.

We will then see how all this influences our **habits** and **behaviours** and finally how our **habits** and **behaviours** influence the **process of disease** in the mouth. We will then find ways to **modify** or **eliminate behaviours and habits** that do not serve our best interests and our health.

With this understanding we will look anew at the common diseases and conditions of the mouth. We will consider each of the common conditions separately. We will consider each of them in the following way:

1. **Understanding broadly the nature of the disease. (What is it?)**

2. **Understanding broadly the disease process. (What does it do?)**

3. **Using the information we have to intercept the process at whatever point it can be accessed. (What can I do about it?)**

We will keep our focus on what the **person** can do to prevent or modify the process. We will not concern ourselves about what the dentist can do. That is for other books. Neither will we concern ourselves with aspects of the process that we cannot modify, e.g. genetic factors. While we accept that these factors contribute to the overall picture they are **irrelevant** to us here because **we cannot influence** them. Simply put, we cannot change our DNA (at least not yet!). **We will concern ourselves only with things that the person herself/himself can change.**

This approach is about personal power in action.

How To Use The Manual

<u>Welcome to simplicity itself.</u>

All too often people complicate things with elaborate descriptions and sometimes the problem then seems even more difficult to overcome. This is unhelpful, and we may end up feeling overwhelmed believing the whole thing is impossible. **So, with this in mind, we intend to focus on *simple* understanding and *simple* methods to deal with problems.**

The solutions we propose involve <u>daily awareness</u> and <u>daily care.</u>

We hope to encourage good habits, which will replace the bad ones over time. Habits are deeply ingrained behaviour patterns and so need time to be replaced.

<u>**There is no hurry.**</u> <u>**There is no deadline.**</u>

Just commit to the process and the rewards will come in time. **<u>Do not be hard or harsh with yourself if you forget.</u>** Simply resolve to start again. In trying to replace good habits for bad ones **there will be a transition time** when both good and bad are present. **Do not be concerned with this.** Simply note that this is part of the changing process.

Encourage yourself frequently by reminding yourself of the benefits that will result when your new strategy is fully in place.

Remember as well that your new habits **benefit your general health** as well - both psychologically and physically.

Being the agent of change for yourself and seeing your strategy develop and come to fruition is a most empowering event showing you that you can accomplish anything easily and successfully with time, willingness, patience and commitment.

Good Luck!

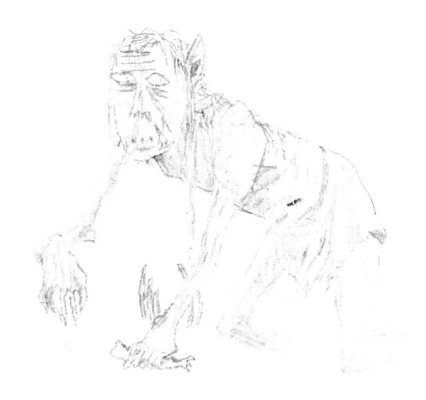

The Mouth is the Mirror of the Body

Look carefully into the Mirror of your Mouth
And the Reflections you behold
Will show you things about yourself
That without your Mirror's gentle help
Would remain hidden and untold.

The gentle light of Understanding
Allows you to appreciate
The simple truth of patterns and rhymes
Ghosts of Guilt from childhood times
That in Forgiveness dissipate

Now can the dark clouds of shame and sadness
Give way to a healed bright mind in gladness.

Philip Christie.

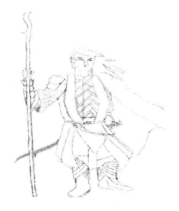

Chapter 1

Do You Mind?

Chapter 1.

Do You Mind?

I think therefore I am ~Rene Descartes

You have been used to looking at things in a certain way. You have assumed that it was the **only** way to look. You have been used to getting things done to your teeth, fillings etc. The focus has always been on the teeth. The focus has always been to get the dentist to find the problems and then get the dentist to fix them.

Now it is time to change the focus. We want to get to the **origin** of the problems so that we may prevent them arising in the first place, - so we can avoid in so far as possible the need for treatment by the dentist.

We will begin by putting the focus on the mind. Your mind may seem a million miles from your teeth and indeed it is, in many ways. But as you begin to see the connection between your mind and your teeth, you will also begin to see what an important connection it really is! You will see as well the enormous potential to you and to your health of understanding this **'Mind Connection'**.

What is mind?

What do we mean by mind?
When we speak about mind in this context we mean ideas, notions, attitudes and beliefs that we hold in our minds as true. They are formed and shaped in childhood in response to situations and experiences. These situations and experiences are shaped by the general context of the society/community into which the child is born. So the prevailing notions, attitudes and beliefs of the society/community and its value systems will have acted as the template for the parents' mindset as the parents' mindset will have acted as the template for the child's.

Some of these ideas, notions, attitudes and beliefs can be quite negative. Some common examples might be **"I am not good enough"**, **"I am not worthy"**, **"I am no good"**, **"I am a failure"**.

These ideas are often formed in the child's mind when a parent reacts in an aggressive or hostile manner to the child's bad behaviour or mistake. The parent, out of frustration, might say things like **"What kind of idiot are you?"** or **"You should be ashamed of yourself!"** or **"Can you do anything right?"**

While the parent means no harm as such, and is acting out of deep frustration or anger, the child takes the parent's word as **ultimate truth.** After all, the parent is the young child's entire world and absolute authority.

The child is often **devastated inside** by the angry words coming from its only source of love, comfort and security.

Little wonder then that the child internalizes the words as true, feeling deeply hurt and believing that he/she is somehow flawed, unworthy, no good or not good enough.

As he thinketh in his heart, so is he...
~ Proverbs 23.7

Psychologists call these ideas and notions 'negative automatic thoughts'. Clearly the ideas and notions are put together by the child's mind and so are not really rational. They often make no sense at all but the child's mind believes them to be true. Maybe some of you have had the experience of trying to convince a child that there are no monsters trying to take him/her away, after the child has had a nightmare. It is not always easy to bring a frightened child around even though what the child thinks makes no sense at all. So the mind can hold onto all sorts of notions and ideas which are held as true although there is absolutely no sense, never mind truth, in them.

Nonetheless these ideas or beliefs are **held** in mind as **true**. But because ideas like these are extremely painful to us, understandably we will always try to avoid them. We do this by burying and hiding them deep in our unconscious minds where they cannot be seen either by ourselves or by anyone else. We figure that will keep us safe and avoid pain. These negative thoughts, ideas, and notions are then **protected** by the very fact of being buried and hidden in the darkness of the unconscious mind.

What is more, these ideas and notions hidden in the unconscious will obviously be brought into adulthood. Yet since they are buried and hidden in the unconscious mind, people will genuinely **not be aware** that these 'negative automatic thoughts' are present in their minds.

Indeed, adults like to think that *they* could not hold wrong ideas and beliefs in their minds. They like to think that they are beyond such childishness. This is not true at all. Adults are quite prone to childishness. How many have not argued bitterly about what movie to go see or some other trivial matter? I know that I have!

So how do you know whether these negative automatic thoughts are hidden in **your** unconscious mind or not?

The simple truth is that they are very likely to be present unless your childhood was perfect with perfect parents.

Frankly, this is impossible unless you were raised on a different planet! Therefore, we can all be sure that we have these 'negative automatic thoughts' to some degree or another.

It is important that we are able to look at ourselves with honesty. This is not always easy but there is immense freedom in it. The thing to remember is that every family will have experienced these patterns. The patterns are, after all, modeled on the accepted notions and ideas of a society and all our mothers and fathers were products of that society. This is simply a matter of fact and not a matter of judgment. There need be no shame in the acknowledgement of patterns into which we were all born.

What a man thinks of himself...determines or rather indicates his fate.
~ Henry David Thoreau

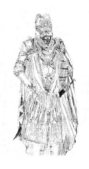

Chapter 2.

Feelings - Nothing More Than Feelings!

Chapter 2
Feelings - Nothing More Than Feelings!

We know too much and feel too little.
~ Bertrand Russell

Out of sight but not out of mind!

Although these ideas are well hidden out of sight, they are still *active* in the unconscious. This means that they still have *effects*. They are held in the mind as *true* and therefore continue to have effects.

Our next task is to follow the pathway of our unconscious negative automatic thoughts and ideas as they produce effects in our feelings and emotions.

It does not take very much to understand this particular step. Obviously, a thought like **"I am not good enough"** is not going to cause you to **feel good** about yourself. Indeed any of the negative thoughts or notions is going to bring on negative feelings.

We will now give some time and space to the connection between our thoughts (what we think) and our feelings.

We find this connection through what is known as "stress".

Seeing's believing, but feeling's the truth
~ Thomas Fuller M.D.

So How Are Your Feelings?

Stress is perhaps the most talked about subject of our modern times. Stress is talked about for very good reason. Levels of stress in modern times have not only affected the quality of our lives but have also contributed in large measure to the deterioration of the quality of our health in general. Stress related illness has fast become the bane of modern living.

It is extremely difficult to define exactly what is stress. Many definitions of stress have been put forward and some have become fashionable. Unfortunately the fashionable ones, usually the most accepted, are often the least accurate.

The most obvious example of this is equating stress with "busyness" or being too busy. However, as everybody knows it is possible to be extremely busy but perfectly at ease with the situation. Indeed, I am sure that we have all been in situations where although we have had a lot to do, we feel happy and content with our lot. In such a situation we are not stressed.

However, we may have a lot to do and **feel very unhappy about it.** Perhaps we feel that others are not doing their share and as such, forcing undue hardship on us. This causes us to feel unhappy and even resentful. This is most definitely stress. Therefore it is not so much the circumstances we find ourselves in, **as how we feel about them.**

We may often blame the circumstances (job, family, etc.) especially when we feel powerless to do anything about them. This can make us feel as though we are trapped. It is this **feeling** of **being trapped** and not being able to do anything (**powerlessness**) about it that is stressful. In these simple examples we get the clue to understanding the **nature of stress**. Stress is about the way you are *feeling*.

It does not matter the circumstances.

You need simply ask yourself **"how do I feel?"** If you do not feel completely at ease, then there is stress present to one degree or another. The greater the feeling of not being at ease the greater is the stress. You can easily imagine the great range of stressful feelings. Consider the **feelings** of mild **annoyance** at finding a queue at the checkout when you are in a hurry. Compare this to the stress of **intense feelings of grief** at the death of a loved one.

Stress has to do with how we are **feeling** and is therefore an expression of our **emotional well being**. Stress then could be said to be any form of negative emotion such as fear, worry, doubt, anxiety, bitterness, regret, annoyance, frustration, resentment, anger, rage, grief etc.

We now have the connection between mind (negative automatic thoughts) and **negative feeling/emotion,** which has become **known as stress**. What we **think** about ourselves (mind) is clearly going to colour how we are **feeling** in any given circumstance. If we think that we are succeeding we will feel good. If we think that we are failures we will feel despair. This is obvious. Therefore our negative notions and ideas about ourselves which we have learned in childhood and which we have hidden in the darkness of the unconscious have major effects on our feelings/emotions.

Our negative automatic thoughts may be hidden out of sight but they continue to affect our feelings, particularly negative feelings. As such they contribute substantially to our stress levels (negative feelings/emotions).

The Trouble With Feelings

Cry baby - Cry baby!

One of the greatest travesties against the person has been society's attitude to crying. The attitude to tears reflects the attitude to feelings, particularly negative feelings, - hurt, sadness, frustration etc. This attitude could be summed up in one word, - **'DENY'**.

Why do we deny? We deny because we think (believe) that admitting them is a sign of weakness, an admission that we are not 'in control'. We are not 'able' not 'strong enough'. We are somehow less than we **ought** to be.

Think a while about the common phrases around tears. "Don't be so foolish" is common. What is this saying except that to cry is to be foolish! And who wants to admit to being foolish?

"Stop that crying" is another all too common phrase. So you are **commanded** to not express your feelings. In this you are made to feel 'wrong' to feel hurt and upset and to give expression to that hurt and upset. Even worse, sometimes this order not to express your hurt is followed by the threat of punishment - "Stop that crying or I will give you something to cry about!"

Even when we try to be nice to the person who is upset, the focus is on trying to make the person stop crying. We might say something like "Now come on, there is no need for that." So now there is **no need** for expressing your feelings.

What about "Don't be such a cry-baby". The implication here is that anyone who cries is behaving like a baby. So now our tears form the basis of a judgment on our level of maturity! Nobody wants to hear that they are immature. Is it any wonder that we deny our feelings?

There is still another most important point that needs to be made here in relation to the way society teaches us to deny our feelings. This relates to gender difference. You see, however bad it is to have feelings, it is much worse to have them if you are male. You are not worthy to be a man or a boy if you cry. "Don't be such a sissy" or "Now you are behaving like a girl" are common. What about "Big boys don't cry" or "You'll have to be a man about this"?

It is quite clear that feelings (barely tolerable in girls and that's just because of their 'weakness') are totally intolerable in boys. In essence it is not acceptable to be what we are - **human**.

Consider the enormous pain inherent in not being able to be what we are. In such a circumstance we will seem to be in a constant but unwinnable battle. How can we achieve the goal of making of ourselves that which we are not? If we realised how much suffering is caused by these totally mistaken attitudes we would be appalled.

Without realising the significance of it, we have denied a most fundamental part of ourselves and this denial has meant that we have trapped ourselves in suffering. We feel hurt and upset but we must not show it. We must keep it to ourselves and keep battling on. How could we be at ease when this constant battle rages within? Worse still, what hope is there when it is not possible to win the battle?

This is something that we must address in relation to stress/negative emotion. We must be free to express ourselves fully, no matter what the emotion. What we get out (express) cannot hurt us further but what we keep inside will torment us and cause suffering.

All emotions are pure which gather you and lift you up: That emotion is impure which seizes only one side of your being and so distorts you.
~Rainer Maria Rilke

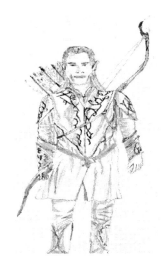

Chapter 3.

To Do Or Not To Do?

Chapter 3.

To Do Or Not To Do?

Habit is either the best of servants or the worst of masters

~ Nathaniel Emmons

The next stage of the story is to understand how stress affects **what we do,** i.e. our habits and behaviours.

What do we mean by behaviours and habits?

These two items are very closely related to each other. **Behaviours** are patterns of **'doing things'** that we set up in our lives. For example, what time we go to bed at night and what time we get up in the morning. **Habits** are more **ingrained patterns** of behaviour and imply **less conscious 'doing'**. An example of this might be smoking. Although we are aware of what we are doing, any smoker will tell you that the cigarette could be in the mouth and lighting before any conscious thought of 'doing it'. Indeed where someone is preoccupied they will often light a cigarette and find that they have one already lighting in the ashtray. This gives some idea of how habits can be relatively unconscious.

But habits can also be so **ingrained** as to be **automatic** without any conscious awareness. This means that a person will genuinely not be aware of what is going on. Nail biting in a child might be a good example here. This child is often startled when someone points out that they are biting the nails. This is because they genuinely did not realize that they had **fallen into** the habit.

When we begin to look at ourselves and our lives we notice all manner of habits and behaviours, which we either did not notice or maybe just did not really think about. As we become observers of ourselves we notice more and more of the complex patterns of habit and behaviour, which make up the tapestry of our daily life. There will be good and bad, negative and positive, helpful and unhelpful and everything in between, making up this intricate tapestry of our individual style.

Making a habit of it!

We will now look at some of the habits and behaviours that have consequences in the mouth and in the various tissues of the mouth. To make it a little easier to understand we will try to think about the mouth as an organ in the body and like all the other organs it has its own jobs to do. The lungs bring life giving oxygen into the blood. The heart must pump the blood around the body. The kidneys filter out impurities from the blood. The mouth as an organ has **two** main jobs or functions.

(a) Eating of food for sustenance.

(b) Speaking for communication.

Either of these two main functions may have negative habits or behaviours associated with them and each of these habits/behaviours will have implications not only for the mouth as a system but also on the body in general. We will then look at **other habits** not directly connected with the mouth but with consequences for the tissues in the mouth.

Habits Related To Eating

When the stomach can't stomach it!

Consider first of all habits/behaviours associated with food and eating. Probably the most obvious habit/behaviour associated with eating is **overeating** or sometimes called **comfort eating.** The term '**comfort eating'** gives the clearest indication of the origin of the problem. Eating for comfort tells us that there is an uncomfortable feeling present that we are attempting to ease (comfort) by eating.

Some people describe this feeling as one of **'emptiness', which** they are trying to fill with food. This **negative feeling** (or stress) is often associated with **poor self-esteem.** The words **'not enough'** or **'never enough'** describe both the emotional feeling and the actual problem with the food. These words may also describe the 'negative automatic thoughts', which are hidden in the unconscious mind. It is very easy to see how the thoughts, feelings and behaviour follow on each other. The behaviour leads to increased weight and loss of shape, which supports and strengthens the original beliefs (not good enough, ugly) and feelings (upset, depression) and the vicious cycle is established.

What are the consequences of overeating?

First of all, rather than producing any comfort (as was the person's intention) the behaviour produces actual physical discomfort. This is the physically uncomfortable feeling in the stomach of being too full. The stomach is over distended or over-stretched. This will produce the pain/discomfort of indigestion. Constant overfilling of the stomach tends to have the effect of pushing part of the stomach up through the muscle wall, which is supposed to contain it. This leads to a condition called 'hiatus hernia' which allows acid from the stomach to come back up the gullet (oesophagus) creating a burning sensation in the chest and throat known commonly as heartburn or acid heartburn (more pain and discomfort).

Overeating is also associated with the tendency (habit) to regurgitate food into the mouth after it has been swallowed into the stomach. The eating disorder bulimia is an extreme and severe condition where a person binges (overeats) and then vomits the food to avoid putting on weight. Such a person needs to be understood. First there is the strong craving for food, which produces the binge eating. This is immediately followed by guilt and the fear of getting fat or fatter. The 'solution' then is to regurgitate or force a vomiting. The less severe habit of regurgitating food into the mouth as a result of overeating, is more common. This regurgitation happens when the stomach is too full and may be brought on by belching due to the pressure within the stomach. Usually the person will swallow the regurgitated food again.

The damage to the teeth is the result of the acid from the stomach being in the mouth where it does not belong. Obviously the damage is proportional to the degree or severity of the condition. This damage is known as **acid erosion** and it is quite common. Mostly the damage is over time and neither noticed nor understood. There may however, be quite severe damage to the teeth in a relatively short time from bulimia and indeed the teeth may become quite sensitive. Tooth damage of this sort is often the first indication of an eating disorder since the sufferer hides the behaviour out of a strong sense of shame.

Sometimes the acid erosion comes from the habit or behaviour of eating very acidic foods. I have met a few people who loved to suck on lemons!

Recent evidence shows that dental erosion is on the increase in young children and teenagers. This appears to be related to the huge increase in the consumption of "fizzy drinks". This could be said to be a societal trend or behaviour. It is fundamentally related to the tendency of parents to "give in" to the child's demand for this type of beverage. The power of television advertising does not help parents control this negative behaviour in their children and points to the need for more integrity from companies producing these beverages. It is wise for parents to realize that it is often 'profit only' that motivates these companies. They are not necessarily concerned with the well being of their young customers or the parents, unfortunately. **Parents be aware!**

Habit is habit, and not to be flung out of the window by any man, but coaxed downstairs a step at a time.
~ Mark Twain

More Stress And More Food Habits!

<u>Sweet Comforts Of Life!</u>
We have seen that the link between stress and dental disease is through our habits and behaviours. While the link between stress and sugar consumption may not be very obvious at first glance, a good look at our behaviours can be very revealing.

Have you ever noticed when a baby cries a lot we often try to calm them with the use of sweet taste. Maybe some of you remember seeing a mother dip a 'soother' or dummy in sugar before putting it in the baby's mouth. The idea is that the sweet taste will soothe the baby and so stop it crying. When we want to get a child to do something we may promise them 'something nice' which is usually a sweet treat.

When we use sugar in this way we set up an association between sugar and comfort and between sugar and reward. These associations are carried into adulthood and may set up varying degrees of negative behavioural patterns with sugar.

A Spoonful Of Sugar Helps The Medicine Go Down!

These behavioural patterns are **mostly unconscious**. We really don't think about it 'like that'. In fact we don't think about it at all. However, for people who have set up associations between sweet taste and comfort, there will be the tendency to increased use of sweet taste when things are not going our way or when we are upset for any reason. If there are things to do which we would rather not do, we might use sweet taste as a reward for getting these things done. The 'negative automatic thought' in this case might be **'my life is so difficult'** or **'I always get the worst deal'** or **'it is not fair'** or **'poor me'**. The perceived bitter pill of life or job or relationship needs to be sweetened to make it acceptable or even tolerable.

This trend is reflected in society in general. A few minutes looking at the adverts on television will show how 'hooked' we are on 'sweet'. Children will often reject anything that is not chocolate flavoured. Even the breakfast cereal must be laced with it! This behaviour will do nothing for the teeth of this generation. In a separate section called "Advice to Parents" we will deal with these issues in more detail.

Sugar frequency in the daily diet (number of times per day) can be seen to be a stress-related behaviour. Our scientific research is clear in identifying **sugar frequency** in the daily diet as the **major factor** in tooth decay. Here again we find the link between stress, behaviour and disease. In human terms we can think of sugar frequency as the tendency we have to feel the need to sweeten our lives or ourselves. Clearly then, when we are upset or not feeling good for whatever reason (stressed) we will have the tendency to **feel** the **need** to sweeten ourselves. The disease of tooth decay (tooth rot) is directly reflecting this stress behaviour.

We first make our habits.
Then our habits make us.
~English Poet

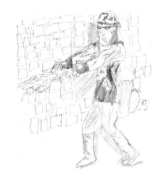

Chapter 4

Speak Your Mind

Chapter 4.

Speak Your Mind

To thine own self be true and it must follow, as the night the day. Thou can'st not then be false to any man..

~ William Shakespeare

Habits Related To Communication

We will devote a full section to explaining this particular habit because its effects are so far reaching and because it is so poorly understood even within the dental profession. We bring together knowledge from dentistry as well as **human understanding** to shed light on this very common yet mostly unconscious habit. I have dubbed it "The keep your mouth shut!" habit.

Keep Your Mouth Shut!

Allow me to introduce what is known in the trade as **bruxism**. A person **squeezes** (**clenches**) and **rubs** (**grinds**) the teeth together. Sometimes it is mainly squeezing the teeth and at other times it is mainly rubbing the teeth. Oftentimes it is a bit of both. These behaviours are really the same habit but with minor variations on a theme. **Most people have this habit** to one degree or another but have no idea that they are doing it. **It is more often than not completely unconscious.**

This can be difficult to understand at first. People think that they would **know** if they had the habit and cannot fathom being told that something is happening that they are not aware of.

The best way to understand this is to recognize how **little** we are aware of body functions. This is because the vast majority of functions in the body are **automatic** and take place without conscious awareness, e.g. breathing, heart rate, blood pressure, liver function, kidney function etc. All of these functions are happening all of the time, - in every second of life but nobody is aware of them.

Therefore it need not come as a surprise to find that habits can also be unconscious.

This very common habit of clenching and grinding the teeth (**bruxism**) can be related to the behaviour (habit) of **'keeping the mouth shut'.** We can all identify to some degree or other with this behaviour. Something happens and we find ourselves upset about it. Maybe someone promised something and did not deliver or someone makes what seems to us to be excessive demands on us or on our time. We want to say something about it but we are afraid. The person may be elderly and we do not want to upset them. We may be afraid that they would think badly of us or would not be friends with us if we spoke. We may be frightened of someone becoming angry or aggressive as a result of what we say. So we decide to keep our mouths firmly shut!

As you can easily imagine such a scenario sets up considerable frustration (stress) within us. Worse still, our choice (behaviour) not to speak ensures that the stress remains inside with no hope of getting out. The more upset and annoyed we are about the situation the greater the stress.

This habit/behaviour could be said to be one which denies the second main function of the mouth system, - communication.

Let's take a good look at how this works. We begin in the mind with the idea that it is 'best' to keep the mouth shut. Maybe we were punished or harshly treated as children when we admitted doing something wrong. Maybe the notion that children should be 'seen and not heard' was upheld by the threat of punishment. How many were smacked or caned at school for 'talking'? The child believes that to 'keep the mouth shut' is best, and will avoid or prevent punishment.

Imagine now that something happens which produces upset in us and we really want to express how we are feeling but we are afraid and stick to the policy of keeping the mouth shut. This makes us feel frustrated and more upset. We are now very stressed.

The most common physical sign of stress is increase in muscle tension.

This increase in muscle tension specifically relates to the large muscles of the jaw, which have been effectively ordered to stay tight and in tension. They obey the order, triggering the habit of clenching and grinding. This increases the pressure in the jaw/muscle system and increases the pressure on all the tissues in the mouth, including teeth and gums. The increases in pressure will be in both the **amount of force** generated (strength) and in the **length of time** for which the force is applied. Simply put, we will exert greater pressure on the system and for longer periods of time.

What are the effects of this habit?

The effects of clenching and grinding are **very wide-ranging**. All of the teeth and the related structures in the jaw/tooth system are affected to one degree or another. This means the possibility of **wear** and **loosening of the teeth** as well as an increased likelihood of **fracture of the teeth**. The **supporting structures** (gum and bone) of the teeth can also be affected and increasing **looseness** can result. Sometimes it is the **jaw joint** (in front of the ear) that is affected resulting in clicking in the joint, locking in the joint and/or pain in the joint.

Sometimes the muscles of the jaw are affected resulting in restricted opening and/or restricted movement. There may be quite severe pain associated with opening and/or movement.

Oftentimes it is a combination of all or many of the above. Generally, one could say that it will be the 'weakest link' in terms of tissue where the greatest problems will arise. This can vary from one case to another. The 'weakest link' tissues are the ones most likely to cause pain or discomfort. For example, if the 'weakest link' were a tooth, - it might fracture causing pain. If the 'weakest link' were gum tissue there might be an increase in bleeding or an increase in looseness and/or tenderness around a particular gum area. We can see therefore that the habit of clenching/grinding can have far reaching effects on the tissues of the mouth and not just on the teeth as you might expect.

We have looked at habits and behaviours that relate to eating and speaking and how they impact on the health of the tissues in the mouth. These habits and behaviours account for the vast majority of disease requiring treatment in the mouth.

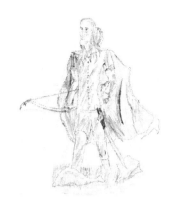

Chapter 5

Other Habits Affecting the Teeth

Chapter 5

Other Habits Affecting The Teeth!

We are what we repeatedly do

~ Aristotle

It is possible for an experienced dentist to tell whether a person is left-handed or right-handed from a simple examination of the teeth. This is because certain brushing habits produce clear evidence of damage and left-handed people produce opposite side damage from right-handed people. It is very simple really!

Scrub-a-dub dub!

This is the habit of over-zealous brushing. People put huge effort into their brushing using hard brushes. I often describe these people as those who "care too much". Unfortunately, the excessive energy that these people put into their effort results in damage.

Many people have grown up listening to parents telling them how important it is to work "hard". This is the measure of a person's worth. How often have you heard the phrase " hard-working man or woman" being used as a way of praising someone? Maybe children were criticized constantly for "not putting enough effort in" or constantly told that they "could do better".

It is easy to see how these ideas can take hold in the child's mind as he/she tries desperately to please Mum or Dad. No effort is ever enough - "I must try harder". "The harder I try, the better I am and the more I will be loved"

"Hard" is understood to be "hard in a physical sense". Effort is equated with physical effort and maybe the perceived harshness of life in general sets the tone for life's daily requirements.

The result is a habit/behaviour of excessive force being used in a genuine attempt to do the job to the highest standard. Unfortunately, this habit is, in fact, counterproductive and results in more damage to the teeth and gums. This increases the amount of treatment needed rather than preventing it.

More habits!

There are still other habits, which will affect the teeth to one degree or another.

Nail biting may produce excessive force on the teeth used for the habit. Biting or chewing pens or pencils is another similar habit. Chewing items of clothing is another variation on the same theme.

Thumb or finger sucking is a well-known habit, which has been associated with dental problems for a long time, often producing conditions, which require braces (Orthodontics) to correct. Thrusting of the tongue may produce similar problems to thumb or finger sucking.

Smoking (another stress habit) has recently been shown to be a risk factor for gum disease.

The main thing to remember with all of these habits is that they are signs of stress in the individual however young that individual may be. Nail biting is a sign of a feeling of insecurity or fear of what might happen. Thumb or finger sucking is clearly a comfort thing, which persists beyond the infant stage.

When these habits/behaviours are understood for what they are, they can be easily remedied. The old way of insisting that the person "Just Stop Doing It!" is a **failed** method. This method will not only always **fail** but will in fact **aggravate** the situation. This is because such a method sees only the unwanted habit and not the factors underneath that support it. This failure to understand cause and effect results in the attempt to change the effect while leaving the cause in place. In fact, the situation gets **worse** because **more stress is created** around the problem.

Imagine a child with a thumb-sucking habit. The issue here is **comfort**. The child is having some difficulty leaving the infant comfort habit behind. The child is afraid to move into the next stage of its development and is resisting the transition. If we just insist he/she stops and maybe even get irritated with the child, then he/she will obviously become even more distressed. Their security is further threatened and the fears are heightened resulting in the need for more comfort from thumb sucking.

The habit is *increased, strengthened* and *supported* by the very attempt to stop it!

It is so important for parents to appreciate this concept. Otherwise they will, even with the very best of intentions, add fuel to the fire and cause the problem to get worse and worse. The more effort they put into **making (forcing)** the child to stop the worse the situation becomes, even to the point of daily conflict between parent and child.

Watch out for substitution!

Another very important consideration with stress habits is that they are interchangeable. If you force a child to stop biting nails they often begin to chew the sleeves of their clothes. If someone forces himself or herself to stop smoking they often begin substituting with other things such as sweet treats. The damage simply moves from lung tissue to tooth tissue.

The habit is not gone.

It has simply been substituted. Many complain that when they give up cigarettes they put on weight. Clearly eating food has become a substitute for cigarette smoking. These substitutions happen when force is used to stop a habit. The person is determined to break a particular stress habit but does not address the underlying problem of stress. All that can happen therefore is substitution and that is not a real change. Be careful of this because what seems to be a "broken" habit is merely a substituted one and this can give a very false impression. This "substitution effect" underlines the need to **deal with the stress** as a priority.

So understanding the origin of the problem (negative ideas in the mind) and how these notions create negative feelings (stress) leading to the physical manifestation of behaviour/habit allows us to deal with the problem effectively. Take thumb-sucking for example. What is actually needed here is **reassurance**. The parent's role is to reassure the child of its safety, thus increasing the child's sense of comfort and security and allowing the child to derive its comfort from the knowledge that **it is always safe** even as it moves into a new phase of development.

This can easily be explained to the child in a way that the child will understand. The habit is understood for what it is and the focus is taken from the actual habit (effect) and placed on the cause (origin). Now and only now is success possible.

There are very serious implications in this understanding. Behaviours and habits will not respond to the old methods of **"make them stop!"** This will simply worsen the problem by adding stress.

The focus must therefore be, - the <u>relief</u> of stress.

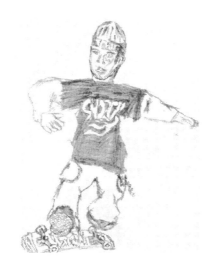

Chapter 6

Putting It All Together

Chapter 6.

Putting It All Together

The Vicious Cycle Of Negative Behavioural Patterns.

This section serves to allow an overview of the entire behavioral machine. The patterns from mind to body can be seen as a never-ending cycle of one thing leading to another and still another, coming all the way around the circle, to begin once again. Indeed, when working in the negative, it could be more aptly described as a descending spiral, with each revolution bringing lower levels of depression and despair.

My message to you, however, is that this spiral can be reversed. It can become an ever-ascending spiral of self-empowerment and confidence in what you can achieve with willingness and commitment. The gentle light of understanding allows clarity with overview and insight. Once seen in this way, the seemingly impossible can give way to hope as solutions dissolve problems.

Follow then the sequence involved -

1. **'Negative automatic thoughts', ideas or notions, learned in childhood and hidden in the unconscious mind -**

lead to

2. Negative feelings/emotional problems, - feelings of being under pressure, - feelings of unworthiness, - feelings of not being good enough, - feelings of not having support, - feelings that life is a bitter pill, etc.

lead to

3. Behavioural patterns or habits generated as a result of these ideas and feelings, e.g. over-eating/comfort eating, - overuse of substances, - sugar, alcohol, tobacco etc. Sometimes these behavioural patterns (habits) can be completely unconscious, e.g. clenching and grinding of the teeth

lead to

4. The production of many physical manifestations, e.g. obesity (overweight) from comfort eating and overeating; dental decay from frequency of sweet (sugar); drunkenness/alcoholism from overuse of alcohol; sinusitis and bronchitis from smoking

lead to

5. The strengthening and reinforcement of the original negative thoughts, ideas and beliefs. The cycle is reinforced and set in motion again as the patterns become more ingrained. Over time these cycles and patterns can seem impossible to break and so

lead to

6. **Attempts to break the habits by force (insisting), which increases the stress and the habit that it supports. This makes the situation worse and the belief that all effort is futile. The feelings of hopelessness and futility, being extremely painful and stressful, add even more fuel to the engine of the habit. The situation now seems impossible.**

The physical results of these behavioural patterns serve to support, reinforce and strengthen the original ideas and feelings. For example, being overweight would seem to support feelings of not being good enough or being ugly. Obviously to have rotted teeth in the mouth, especially if they were visible, would seem to support similar feelings. Gum disease with bleeding (as well as producing a nasty taste and smell) could engender feelings of shame and guilt in the same way.

The 'vicious cycle' nature of these patterns supports, reinforces and strengthens the original thoughts and feelings, which support reinforce and strengthen the behaviours, which support reinforce and strengthen the physical results of the patterns. The cycle sets itself up, reinforces and strengthens itself while it recreates itself anew. The cycle or pattern once established would seem to be very resistant to change.

Round and round it goes, seeming to get stronger with every cycle. It seems so difficult. We wonder where to even begin. This is because circles or cycles have no obvious beginning and so it is that there is no obvious starting point. So where then can we begin?

The beginning of a habit is like an invisible thread but every time we repeat the act we strengthen the strand, add to it another filament, until it becomes a great cable and binds us irrevocably, thought and act.
~ Orison Swett Marden

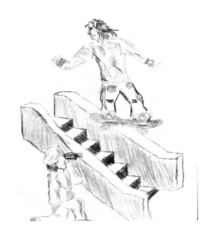

Chapter 7

Where Do I Begin?

Chapter 7.
Where Do I Begin?

A tree as great as a man's embrace springs from a small shoot. A terrace nine stories high begins with a pile of earth. A journey of a thousand miles starts with the first step.

~ Lao-Tsu, Tao Te Ching

At this stage we have travelled from mind (thoughts) through feelings and stress (emotions), to behaviours and habits which have effects in the body. We have established the MIND/BODY connection in clear and easy steps.

Our next mission is to use this new light of understanding to access the process at each of the different levels that we have identified, in order to make practical use of each one.

Minding Yourself!

We begin with mind. How can we cause changes in these 'negative automatic thoughts'. The first thing to appreciate is that **changing the mind is NOT easy.** It *sounds* easy but **it is not**. The reason is that ideas and notions like these are deeply rooted and established since childhood.

Secondly, they hide in the unconscious mind and therefore, as far as a lot of people are concerned, they do not even exist!

The simplest technique for mind change is the use of affirmations. Maybe some of you will have come across Louise Hay's book "You Can Heal Your Life". In this excellent book Louise shows us the effects on our health of negative thoughts, ideas and notions. She recommends positive affirmations to replace the negative ideas.

The biggest problem with positive affirmations is that **belief is lacking** in the words you are using. This means that people complain that it sounds stupid and they feel stupid saying it. It is little wonder then that they tend to give up on the effort.

Simply telling people that this will happen and to expect it is an enormous help.

They now know that it is something everyone experiences with affirmations and not something they are doing wrong. This makes it more likely that they will continue with daily affirmations long enough for it to make a difference.

The other way to change the mind is through therapy or counselling with a professional counsellor or therapist. This is particularly good when problems seem resistant to change. Obviously choose a therapist with care and make sure that you are comfortable with your chosen therapist and the methods that they use. My own recommendation (from my own experience) is to choose a warm and human therapist rather than the cold analytical one.

If you are distressed by anything external, the pain is not due to the thing itself but to your own estimate of it; and this you have the power to revoke at any moment.

~ Marcus Aurelius

Keep the daily affirmations short and sweet and to the point. It should take less than a minute so that you can repeat them to yourself hourly (if possible). Use only the present tense. For example, say:

I am always good enough
I am good
I am loving
I am lovable
I am worthy
I am deserving

If you notice a little voice in you saying, " This is nonsense! It won't do any good." do not be in the slightest concerned. Simply reply " I have to give things a chance before passing judgment. How can I know that it is nonsense and will not work if I have not tried it?"

Stress management!

The next task is to deal with negative feelings. This is what has become known as **stress management** and there is an absolute wealth of programmes available these days to choose from.

Use the one that appeals to you.

The scientists call it biofeedback or autogenic training. The medical people call it the parasympathetic (relaxation) response. Others call it Yoga while still others call it Transcendental Meditation. **It really does not matter what you call it**.

It would be very worthwhile indeed to investigate one, if not all, of the various approaches which I have mentioned above. When you find one that "suits" you, one that resonates with you and you are comfortable with it, you have truly found a treasure.

The various techniques have in common the goal of deep relaxation, what one might call an increasingly profound stillness or sense of being **'at ease'**. This is a skill that anyone can learn because everybody is 'wired for it'. This means that everybody has the biological mechanisms that make it possible. Like any skill it is developed by practice, daily practice.

Developing the skill of being calm and at ease

Stress is about how we are 'feeling'. We have defined stress as negative feeling/emotion. Therefore what we want to do in order to deal with stress is to minimize negative feelings while maximizing positive feelings. The best way of achieving this is to learn the art of deep relaxation. This is a skill that **needs to be learned**. Like any skill it must be practiced regularly in order to develop the skill and master it.

Therefore the practice of deep relaxation should become a daily ritual.

According to the experts in this field, twenty minutes twice a day will be enough to begin to develop the skill. This skill takes time to master. Again the experts say that a person will need 30-70 days consistent and diligent practice before they will notice a difference. As we continue with daily practice we begin to notice that we feel more and more at peace.

People sometimes complain that they don't have time to give 20mins. twice a day. Think what this must mean! When we say this, we are saying that we don't have time for our health and well being. Imagine if someone said that they did not have time to eat! We would immediately say how crazy that idea is! Be assured that deep relaxation really is as important to health as eating!

There is nothing training cannot do. Nothing is above its reach. ~ Mark Twain

The people who think they don't have time for this are those most in need of it!

When we first begin to practice, we are often horrified to realize how stressed we really are. This is perfectly normal.

Do not in any way be put off by this. Everybody will experience this problem.

If anyone out there thinks they have no stress, - think again!! There are very few indeed who are stress free. Anyone who is stress-free has been practicing deep relaxation for years.

Another common misunderstanding made at the beginning is that a person thinks he/she must be **"doing it wrong"**. People think this all the time but the good news is that it is almost impossible to do it wrong. Sometimes people decide to stop because they think it is 'not working'.

It is very important to understand that deep relaxation works at the level of the unconscious mind and therefore it is not possible to 'know' in the conscious mind whether it is working or not.

The answer then is simple. Choose a method, which appeals to you, and commit to practicing diligently and consistently. Do not try to figure out whether or not it is working or how well you are doing. Just keep practicing daily and you will see the results in time. Patience and consistency will bring the rewards.

The only mistake that anyone can make is to give up!

You will notice with time that your mind is increasingly calm and peaceful. When problems arise you will deal better with them. You will notice that problems upset you less than before and solutions to them come to mind easier and easier.

As you begin to master the skill of deep relaxation, you become more and more 'stress-hardy'. This means that things and situations, which used to make you feel hurt and upset, no longer affect you in that way.

Obviously, this will mean a **very real loosening of the hold of the habits and behaviours,** which seemed so resistant before. This happens because the habits and behaviours are supported and strengthened by stress and when the stress diminishes, the support and strength of habits and behaviours also diminishes.

When we bring the light of understanding to the habits and behaviours, while at the same time continuously and consistently reducing the stress by daily practice, the deep roots of our negative behavioural patterns and habits are more easily shaken loose. We are then begining to reclaim our power over them.

Things do not change, we change
~ Henry David Thoreau

To Do Or Not To Do! --- Dealing with the behaviours.

So far we have tried to tackle the thoughts in the mind and most importantly embarked on a course of daily stress management. These are necessary requirements and must be in place **before** tackling the actual behaviours. It is also wise to remember that there may be a transition period where both the old behaviours and habits are still present even though we are working to bring in the new. Again do not be in the slightest concerned about this. **It is part of the process of change.** As the new methods become more and more established, so the old habits, no longer hidden and supported, fall away easily in time.

The habit engine

It is useful to imagine habits as engines, which use stress as fuel. If we **try to stop the engine** but **continue to supply the fuel** we are defeating our own purpose. We are, in fact, **supporting the habit and trying to stop it at the same time.** The result is **effort wasted** and **no result!** It is like trying to apply the brakes on the bicycle and peddling harder at the same time.

This is the primary reason why people put great effort into trying to change habits but consistently fail. How many people have put great effort into giving up cigarettes only to go back smoking again? How many times have you heard people say that they have tried and tried to give up cigarettes but always failed. They quite **understandably** conclude that they are **not able** to stop!

The good news is that the person's ability is not the problem. They simply have not given themselves a chance. What hope has anyone to stop the habit machine when there is as much or more energy keeping it going as there is trying to stop?

The solution is to **close off the fuel supply to the habit engine.** This is done by simply committing to the daily practice of stress management (deep relaxation). As the fuel for the habit engine runs dry, the habit easily falls away with little effort. This same concept can be applied to any habit no matter how ingrained.

So if you have ever despaired of breaking habits, from alcohol and cigarettes to nail biting and pen chewing, - take heart!

The answer is here, simple and inexpensive and yours for the taking!
It is also good to know that you **can** succeed!

Every effort is a success in that it brings you closer to your goal!

There is nothing so disempowering as the thought of not being able to change, despite your best efforts. Indeed this can result in feelings of hopelessness and despair, which generate the most horrible of psychological suffering.

Great news then, there is nothing wrong with you. You had simply set yourself the impossible task of stopping and starting at the same time! Your new method of cutting off the fuel supply to the habit engine **will** bring results in time.

So what action is needed?
At this stage we have brought the gentle light of understanding to the unconscious mind where we have found some of our negative automatic thoughts, ideas and

notions about ourselves. This gentle light has allowed us to understand the origin and nature of those thoughts. It has also allowed us to realize that they are **not true**. They are related to a **child's view** of difficult childhood experiences and formed around much hurt, pain and upset. This understanding allows us, maybe a little laugh at the thoughts that have caused us so much pain over the years.

We have also committed to dealing with the negative feelings (emotions) associated with the negative thoughts with daily practice of deep relaxation. We have begun the process of making ourselves stress-hardy. **All that remains to do now is to make decisions. We use our power of choice to change and modify those habits and behaviours, which are not serving our best interests.**

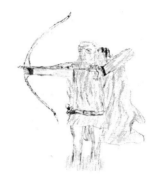

Chapter 8

Preventing Tooth Decay And The Need For Fillings

Chapter 8.

Preventing Tooth Decay And The Need For Fillings

There is nothing training cannot do. Nothing is above its reach. It can turn bad morals to good; it can destroy bad principles and recreate good ones; it can lift men to angelship. ~ Mark Twain

We are now ready to make very practical use of the understanding that we have gained so far. We are going to prevent the need for any future fillings by simply making a choice (decision) to modify (change slightly) a behaviour (habit).

What is tooth decay?

Tooth decay is a disease process, which softens and destroys the hard tissues of the tooth. These tissues are called enamel and dentine. Bacteria, acting on sugar, produce the acid that fuels the disease process.

It is treated by the removal of the rotted (decayed) parts of the tooth and the replacement of the missing parts with a 'filling'.

We have shown a direct relationship between stress and tooth decay. Stress (feeling upset) leads to an increased desire to sweeten our lives and ourselves. This results in a greater **frequency** of sugar in the diet. The increased frequency of sugar in the diet leads to tooth decay.

It is true that there are many other factors in tooth decay, but this is the major factor and one over which we have direct control.

What action do we need to take?

Simply put, the problem is the over-use of sugar (sweet things) in the diet. We have, in our highly stressed modern society, developed the habit of sweetening ourselves too often! This we now realize is a stress habit.

- **Firstly, recognize the role of mind and begin dealing with it as outlined in "Minding yourself" in the previous section.**

- Secondly, start on a course of stress management as outlined in "Stress management" in the previous section.

These two items are common to all the conditions that we will deal with. They should be seen as fundamental requirements, crucially important in helping to **loosen** the **grip** of habits (cut off the fuel supply) and so making modifications in behaviours or habits so much easier to achieve.

What's Next?

The good news is that you **do not** need to ***give up anything!!***

The problem is ***frequency*** or ***the* number of times** per day that sweet things are placed in the mouth. So we **deal** with the frequency.

The **simple secret** is to make a choice (decision) to leave **3.5 to 4** hours between sweet consumptions. Immediately the frequency is reduced to 4-5 maximum per day. It also means that the teeth have this time (4 hours) to **recover** from the effects of acid produced by sugars.

The teeth are then fully recovered before the next acid attack.

Fair Play To You And Your Teeth

This is how I advise my patients. I like to keep it simple and easily understandable. People appreciate ease and simplicity in a seemingly ever more complex world. The simpler the requirements, the more the likelihood of success with more people.

People also readily understand the need for a break for the tissues. After all everybody needs a break!

We call this method "Fair Play To You And Your Teeth" because you **get what you want** and your teeth **get what they want!** It is fair and even-handed.

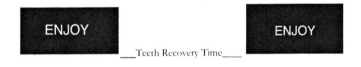

Have what you want!---3.5 - 4 hour break---Have what you want!

If you feel that you must eat something in the ***Recovery Time*** ensure that it is ***sugar-free.***

This strategy has been shown to produce results over as little as 15 weeks.

What do you get for the work you put in?

The benefits of this simple preventive strategy to you are enormous and long lasting.

Direct benefits to your teeth

- Early cavities (those in the earliest stage of disease, sometimes referred to as sticky fissures) literally fix themselves! The softening enamel rehardens itself (**remineralizes)** over time and so **does not need any treatment**--this saves you both **time** and **money**.

- Middle-sized cavities (these are bigger and easier to see or detect) demonstrate that the disease process is slowing over time. They are said to **arrest** (stop) and *may not* require treatment, although a lot of people want larger cavities treated, especially when visible.

- Even with the larger cavities the **disease process slows down** and in time could reasonably be **expected** to **completely arrest**. These large cavities could take 30-40 weeks to completely arrest depending on size. Once again people may want these larger cavities treated especially where they are visible.

Direct benefits to you

- The overall effect could be described as **"putting out the fire of the disease completely"** leaving the person to decide, when and how much rebuilding they want to engage in.

- The **urgency is taken out** of treatment (unless there is pain).

- You take **control of your own situation** and are therefore **empowered.** At the same time help is always available from your dentist if needed.

- Because the disease is under control **pain is less likely** to occur.

- <u>Cost</u> of required treatment is **drastically reduced.**

- <u>Cost</u> of future treatment is **drastically reduced.**

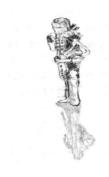

Chapter 9

Preventing Gum Disease

Chapter 9.

Preventing Gum Disease

What is Gum Disease?

Gum disease might be better called **"tooth support disease"** because it breaks down and **destroys** the **supporting tissues** of the teeth. The teeth become loose and sore and either fall out or have to be taken out because of pain. Many older people remember "Pyorrhea" as the name that was used for Gum Disease. Nowadays the name "Periodontitis" or "Periodontal Disease" is preferred.

What causes Gum Disease?

There are many factors at play in Gum Disease. We will talk **only** about those factors over which we have some control.

- **1. Build-up of bacterial plaque around the gums.** This has to do with the **quality** of brushing.

- **2. Breakdown of the natural defenses** of the gum tissue. This has to do with the very complex issue of the defense system (immune system) of the body.

What can you do about it?

- 1. **Prevent the build-up of bacteria around the gum.**

This involves putting more **care** into the **quality** of your brushing. It means **taking more time.** It means having <u>**good method and technique.**</u> It means being careful and thorough. It means giving <u>extra attention</u> to more <u>awkward places</u>. We will devote a full section to Quality Brushing.

- 2. **Prevent or reduce excessive loading on the supporting gum tissue.**

The idea here is to **reduce** the **pressure** on the system as a whole thereby **reducing the strain or loading on the local gum defense (immune) system.** This involves becoming aware of the habit of clenching and grinding of the teeth. This is the Bruxism habit that we have discussed under "Habits related to communication". As you will remember, this habit is **unconscious** with most people and therefore most people are not aware that they do it. **Indeed some people will insist that they don't.** The best way is to go with the evidence. If the evidence is there - then the habit is there. Once again we will devote a full section to "Dealing with clenching/grinding (bruxism)"

Quality Brushing

The requirements for **Quality Brushing** are the **same** as the requirements for doing any job well. You need to know what you are trying to achieve and then to employ the best means for achieving your goal. **Don't be in a hurry** to get it done because this will mean cutting corners and making mistakes.
Slow down - do it well and you can then forget about it until tomorrow.

- **One Quality Brushing per day is more than adequate.**

Your mission is to remove a **soft sticky deposit** (called Bacterial Plaque) from every surface of every tooth. This **plaque is soft and easy to remove.** You may have removed it with your nail at some time or other. If it does not come away easily, it is not plaque. Such a hard deposit is tartar, also known as calculus, and no amount of brushing will remove it. It requires professional cleaning (scaling) to remove it.

The brush is NOT the most important item.
The **person** holding the brush is the **crucial factor.** Do not be fooled by clever advertising and marketing - no brush, no matter what make, can ever be better than the person using it. **A good car does not make a good driver.** Always remember it is the **person** holding the brush **rather** than the **brush** itself. Having said that, use the best quality brush you can afford.

Toothpaste is NOT a major item.

It is only an aid to cleaning. Cleaning can be done without it but it is a good help. As soap is to washing, so toothpaste is to tooth cleaning. It is not essential, but like soap, makes cleaning easier.

So how do you do it?

Use a **soft** toothbrush with a **pea-sized** blob of toothpaste.

Good Method - The Bus Route Rule

Use a **specific direction** for cleaning and stick to it. I call this the **'Bus Route Rule'**. This means always **starting** in the **same place** and always **finishing** in the same place with the **direction in between always the same** - just like the bus.

Good Technique - Focus On The Gum

This **involves** putting the **focus** of cleaning on a **little ditch** called the **sulcus,** which is situated between the tooth and the gum around each tooth. This little ditch is the place where **Gum Disease begins.**

Because **Quality Brushing** is focused on the **prevention** of **Gum Disease**, the brush is angled at a **45°** (degree) **angle** to the gum (into the little ditch). Obviously, this is **45° upwards** for the **upper** teeth and **45° downwards** for the **lower** teeth.

The movement of the brush should be a **backwards and forwards vibration** ↔ or **short circular movements** (similar to the cleaning action of a washing machine). <u>**No scrubbing please**</u> - this can cause damage to both gum tissue and tooth tissue and should be avoided. (See section on Toothbrush Damage).

The Bus-Route Rule

- **If you are right-handed** - Begin the brush journey on the <u>**upper left**</u> **INSIDE** (palate side) at the very back. We begin on the **INSIDES** because they are **often forgotten** and are slightly **more awkward** to do. In this way, we get the harder part of the job done first.

- The brush travels from here <u>**around to the upper right**</u> **INSIDE**. Now drop down to the **lower right INSIDE** and continue around the **lower INSIDE** to the very back of the lower left. We have now **completed** all the **INSIDE** surfaces.

- Next bring your brush over that last tooth on the **lower left** to the **OUTSIDE** and begin to work your way along the **OUTSIDE** surfaces of the lower teeth, coming around to the **lower right.**

- Now move straight upstairs to the **upper right** and move around the **OUTSIDES** of the teeth to the **OUTSIDE** of the **upper left** where you began.

- **If you are left handed** - Begin on the **upper right INSIDES** and follow the reverse course finishing on the upper right **OUTSIDES**.

The important thing is that whatever **method** you choose **stick to it**. If the bus (Brush) always goes in the same direction then you are unlikely to miss some areas while doing others twice. This means that you can be certain that every surface of every tooth has been cleaned. This eliminates the guesswork and you can be sure of **a job well done**.

Especially difficult or awkward areas should receive extra attention, as should those areas more prone to disease (bleeding). These are different for different individuals so you will need to consult your own dentist.

You now have all you need -
- **Plenty of time**
- **Soft Brush** (+ Pea sized blob of tooth-paste)
- **Focused Technique** (45° Angle into the little ditch - with vibration or short circular movements)
- **Definite Method** (Bus Route Rule - **every** surface of **every** tooth!)

Dealing with Clenching/Grinding (Bruxism)

What is Clenching/Grinding?

Clenching/Grinding is the **unconscious habit** of **squeezing** and **rubbing** the teeth together.

It is unconscious and most people will be **totally unaware** of it.

Many people are surprised that this habit can be going on without their knowledge. To understand this, one has to understand that **most of the body functions are unconscious,** e.g. Breathing, Heart Rate, Lung Function, Liver Function, Temperature Regulation etc. In fact, it has been estimated that the body must perform **6 trillion biochemical reactions per second, every second, to sustain life**. All of these are totally unconscious and automatic. The habit of clenching/ grinding is simply another unconscious and automatic happening. Unlike other important body functions, which we have mentioned, the habit of **clenching/grinding is a destructive habit** and so the requirement is to **minimize,** or better still, with time, **eliminate** it altogether.

What can you do about it?

Understanding the problem

We have already seen the nature of this habit as a "keep your mouth shut" policy, which is supported by the notion that it is fearful or dangerous to open the mouth. This can be thought of in much the same way as a computer programme. The notion is programmed into the unconscious mind as a result of the child's experiences at home or at school or both. As a result, there is a blocking of expression (communication) and this leads to much frustration and anger, which remain hidden. Both of these are powerful emotions and can cause tremendous damage if bottled up inside.

The first thing to do is to challenge the notion that keeping your mouth shut is a good policy. Understanding the damage that can result both emotionally and physically is a good place to begin that challenge. Realizing the childhood origin is also helpful. Should a policy decided upon by a child's frightened mind hold sway in the adult's world?

Shakespeare, whose wisdom is as relevant today as it was in his time, advised us on the important principle of speaking our minds (to thine own self be true). So we begin to understand that the danger (problem) is in **not speaking** our minds.

Many say that conflict would result if they spoke out. I can certainly understand this fear. My answer is that it depends on how you say it! Certainly if one confronts another in anger (with all guns blazing), then one cannot expect but a similar reaction from the other person. The result will be further conflict and difficulty. However, if you invite the other person to a calm discussion over a cup of tea or coffee, explaining your difficulties and your feelings, a mutually acceptable result is much more likely to occur.

From the perspective of mind a person would do well to promise oneself "If I have something to say, I will say it!" The saying of it need not be aggressive or pushy but a calm statement of what you think or how you feel.

A stress management programme to deal with emotional issues (negative feelings) is **always** a basic requirement for **loosening** habits/behaviours which are supported by stress.

From a practical point of view, once your dentist has identified the habit, your main task is to bring the habit to your conscious awareness. Remember that most people are not aware that they have the habit.

Awareness of the problem

The best way to start improving the awareness is to simply say to yourself, ***"My teeth should not be together except when I'm eating"***. Then watch out for times when you catch yourself squeezing or rubbing the teeth together. When you notice, **very gently** remind yourself to let go. Don't get upset with yourself when you notice, simply take the mental attitude ***"the more I spot, the more I stop"*** and have the feeling of "I'm glad I noticed, this means it is working". Remember - **SPOTTING IS STOPING.**

Reprogramming your unconscious mind.

I often suggest this method to people who are not keen to spend a lot of time and money doing stress management courses. It is simple and effective and low-cost. However, I would point out that many people (myself included) do better when working with another's help rather than when working alone. Even so, simple self-driven methods can be used to begin the process and other more in-depth methods can follow as greater skill and mastery is acquired.

Although reprogramming your unconscious mind sounds difficult, in fact, it is very easy indeed. All you need do is to **buy yourself some relaxation tapes or CD's** and **commit** to using them for **20mins. before sleeping.** (A second 20min. session during the day would be even better.) These tapes are easily available in good bookstores and health food stores. Choose the ones that appeal to you. It is a good idea to buy three or four different tapes (CD's) so that you don't get bored or fed up with one. Perhaps you could alternate them every three or four days.

The commitment to using them is all you need. Don't try to figure out what's happening or whether it's working or not. Remember the conscious mind is not really involved at all. Simply put your tape on and experience it. Let it wash over you so to speak.

What is actually happening is that, without your knowing, <u>**your brain-wave patterns are changing to more relaxed forms**</u>. This causes a reduction in muscle tension. The reduction in muscle tension reduces tension in the jaws. The reduced tension in the jaws reduces the **habit of clenching and grinding.**

This is not a quick fix method. It requires time and commitment. It can take 30 - 70 days for noticeable change to occur. Your patience will pay off. The only mistake you can make is to give up. Remember you are learning a skill and learning a skill takes time. In many ways it is like learning to play a musical instrument. Commitment, patience and time bring the rewards.

There are many other proven benefits of this type of deep relaxation, not the least of which is a better quality night's sleep. And all of us could benefit from that!

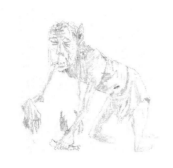

Chapter 10

Joint And Muscle Problems In The Jaw

Chapter 10.

Joint and Muscle Problems in the Jaw
(TMJ syndrome)

What is it?

This is often called TMJ or CMJ syndrome. TMJ (temporomandibular joint) refers to the main jaw joint which is located just in front of the ear-hole. If you place your fingers in this area and move your jaw you will feel the joint moving under your fingers. CMJ (craniomandibular joint) is simply another name for the same joint.

All joints have muscles associated with them to provide movement to the joint. When pain and other symptoms occur in these structures of the jaw it is often called TMJ syndrome. There may be headache associated with this that is often confused with migraine headache.

What are the symptoms?

Pain is not a common feature. Only about 5% of people with joint/muscle problems present with pain. When pain is present it can be very severe, extending from the temple (side of the head) through the joint (in front of the ear) and even into the muscles of the neck. There may be difficulty in opening the mouth and sometimes the jaw is locked and opening is very limited and very painful. Clicking in the joint on opening and closing or on side-to-side movement is very common. This is often present even when there is no pain.

What causes it?

When the joint/muscle system is subjected to excessive force, obviously damage can result. This can happen as a result of an accident or much more commonly as a result of excessive force from the habit of clenching/grinding (Bruxism). Sometimes there may be a little of both involved.

Where the problem has resulted from trauma (accident) recovery will happen in time. Sometimes pain relief is necessary when the condition is acute and an anti-inflammatory medicine is usually the best bet for temporary relief. A dental splint, which is akin to a cast on a broken or sprained arm or leg, may also be helpful in protecting the tissues while they recover.

What can you do about it?

The best preventative approach to this problem (as outlined in the chapter on dealing with clenching/grinding) is to recognize the effects of stress on the mouth and jaw system and to take steps to minimize the problem.

Very simply, note that the habit of clenching/grinding is a stress habit brought on by the policy of "keeping your mouth shut" and decide to take the necessary steps.

1. Revise the "keep your mouth shut" policy to an "open your mouth" policy. Courses in assertiveness can be very helpful in difficult situations. Recognize the origin of the policy as a childhood decision, which has no place in the adult mind.

2. Begin and commit to the stress management course of your choice.

3. Try to increase and maintain your conscious awareness of the habit. "My teeth should not be together, - except when I am eating".

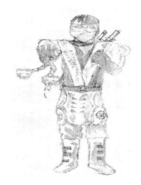

Chapter 11

Tooth Brush Damage

Chapter 11.

Toothbrush Damage

<u>What is it?</u>

Toothbrush damage is known in the trade **as toothbrush abrasion** and is the damage to teeth and gums that results from the use of **excessive force** in brushing, usually using a hard toothbrush. In a way this is the condition of people who **care too much.** Somehow they get to think that unless they really go at it with gusto they won't do a good job. This is a kind of over-zealous enthusiasm where the excess energy actually becomes destructive. We have seen that the idea of always striving to do better, coming from childhood experiences of "you can do better than that!" is at the root of the problem. The genuine desire to do the best is pushed over the top to become over-zealousness.

<u>What is the problem?</u>

The problem is the way in which a person **thinks** about what **is required** in brushing. Somehow people form the **idea** that the job is **very difficult** and **great effort** is required. **This is not true at all.** Plaque is a very soft material, which builds up on the teeth. It is **very soft** and **very easy to remove.**

The problem is therefore very simply a **wrong notion or idea** which leads to **an 'aggressive' approach** to cleaning, **resulting in damage** to **tooth** and **gum** tissue.

How does it affect the teeth?

Toothbrush abrasion affects both teeth and gums. Often the earliest sign of the problem is what people describe as a 'little ledge' in the tooth at the very margin of the gum. The person often feels this with a fingernail and sometimes there is an 'electric shock sensation' when the area is touched with the fingernail or a toothbrush bristle. Very often there are no shocking symptoms although sensitivity to cold is a quite common feature.

As the damage progresses it becomes more and more noticeable, with the gum tissue receding back causing the tooth to look longer as more of its root surface is exposed. Some people refer to this as getting long in the tooth implying that the damage to the tissues is the result of getting older. This is not true! It is related to time only in that the longer the habit persists the greater the damage that occurs.

The damage to the tooth eventually manifests as a v-shaped notch at the gum margin which increases over time both in width and depth. In extreme cases an exposure to the pulp (the living part of tooth at the central core) may happen, or sometimes a fracture of the crown of the tooth may happen due to the increasing weakness of the structure.

What is the solution?

We simply need to change the way we **think** about brushing.

Instead of thinking -
This job is difficult to do -
I need an aggressive approach -
There is harsh action needed -
I need a good hard brush -

Think instead -
This job is	**EASY -**
I will be	**GENTLE with a SOFT BRUSH -**
I will	**TAKE MY TIME -**
I will be	**THOROUGH -**
I will	**NEVER use a HARD BRUSH.**

This change of mind coupled with the change of behaviour and a soft brush is all you need to prevent toothbrush damage.

The solution could not be easier!!

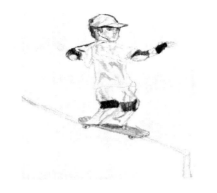

Chapter 12

Acid Damage

Chapter 12.

Acid Damage

What is it?

Acid damage (known in the trade as acid erosion) is the damage that happens to teeth as a result of the action of acid on them.

Where does this acid come from?

The acid can come from either of two sources -

1. **Inside the person - Stomach.**

2. **Outside the person - food or drink.**

Of these two the most **likely** is the **stomach**.

What does it do?

The acid 'corrodes' the enamel and dentine where it comes in contact with them. This shows as corrosive wear marks on the teeth. Enamel (the outer layer or surface layer of the tooth) 'corrodes' with acid at a slower rate than dentine (the layer underneath the enamel). This gives the characteristic 'wear' marks associated with acid erosion.

Fractures of the enamel edge are common making teeth look 'edgy' and a person's appearance is affected. There is seldom any pain although sensitivity to hot and cold may be present. Sensitivity itself is not common with acid erosion. However, when **erosion is rapidly progressive** as a result of bulimia, sensitivity can indeed be a major feature.

When acid erosion occurs **in conjunction** with the clenching/grinding habit the wear on the teeth can be much more severe. Two problems combine to aid and abet each other, so to speak, increasing the severity of the damage produced.

What can you do about it?

We have two sources of acid with which to deal. Although these sources are separate, they are related. You could say that both are 'eating' problems. One has to do with the type of foods (acidic) that we put into the mouth, as well as how much and how often. The other relates to the regurgitation of acid from the stomach into the mouth. Indigestion, heartburn and regurgitation follow after the consumption of food. In this way, it is easy to see the problem as food-related or more correctly 'eating-related'.

1. Modify the acid intake in the diet

Notice the tendency to use acidic foods and make a decision to restrict intake. Some common drinks on the market can be very corrosive. Apparently you can clean old coins in a certain well-known fizzy drink. If it has this effect on metal you can easily imagine the effects on the tooth structure not to mention the effects on the soft tissues.

2. Take steps to ensure the health of the stomach.

Have the stomach checked by your doctor to see if there are any abnormalities present and have whatever treatment is necessary. Be aware of bad eating habits and resolve to change them. Examine this checklist and make your resolutions. It is not difficult to understand the childhood origin of many of these eating habits. How many can remember being told to "Hurry up and finish that dinner!" or "You won't leave that table until the dinner is all gone"

(a) **Never rush your meal - ensure adequate time for eating, chewing and some time afterwards for digestion.**

(b) **Never put food into the mouth while there is food still being chewed. Always wait until one piece of food is swallowed before placing another piece in the mouth.**

(c) **Eat mindfully getting maximum taste and enjoyment from the food.**

(d) Stop when you feel you are full. Do not try to finish everything on your plate. Try not to feel over-full after the meal. Make sure you stop eating before this happens.

These very simple measures can have very significant effects over time. Indeed, some experts say that simple measures such as these will correct any problem relationship with food over time and result in the normalization of weight, whether the problem is being overweight or being underweight.

3. Check for underlying emotional/psychological difficulties.

It is well accepted and understood that eating difficulties often have an emotional or psychological basis. You may for example have heard of 'comfort eating' where a person tends to over-eat when they are upset. This behaviour is very common. When emotional upsets happen the person goes straight to the fridge for the tub of ice-cream. We often see this dramatized on television programmes.

When the **eating patterns** seem to be **resistant** to change, it is then often **worthwhile** to get **professional advice and help.** Exploring this area with an appropriate professional can yield tremendous results. Do not be in any way shy about contacting a **psychologist** or **counsellor** to help you in this. The help and advice that you get will often last a lifetime!

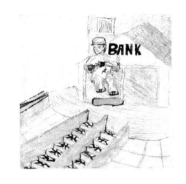

Chapter 13

Prevention For Children

Chapter 13.
Prevention for Children

Teach these things not with your words but with your actions; not with discussion but with demonstration. For it is what you do that your children will emulate, and how you are that they will become.

~ Neale Donald Walshe

First and foremost prevention for children involves the parents in the biggest way. Over the years I have heard parents say to the children when they were with me in the surgery, " I hope you are listening to what the dentist is saying". I often found this frustrating as I addressed the parent and **not** the child. It was clear to me that if there was going to be a change of policy, it would be the parents and not the child that would bring about the initial change.

The child was in fact being asked to behave as the adult and to take adult responsibility when that was clearly impossible. This gives us our first principle.

Parents are the guardians of health in children.

We have already seen that negative thoughts lead to stress and stress supports negative habits. Parents, having taken control of their own stress and understanding how easily we can negatively influence our children (remember that's how we developed our own habits) are now in a good position to guide the children into a stress-free lifestyle. Feeling more at ease within ourselves we are less likely to fly off the handle or make unhelpful remarks at the child when confronted with problems and difficulties. We are then less likely to induce negative thoughts and feelings in the easily impressionable child's mind.

From the point of view of dental disease, the really important issues are:

1. Communication

Teaching the child to always express (**allow out, let out**) feelings and emotions. This is done by allowing the child a safe and loving space for even the most negative of feelings, e.g. frustration, anger or rage.

2. Eating habits

It is important to teach the child good dietary practice and to maintain **parental stewardship** of the dietary content and pattern.

The very best advice that anyone can give parents is that 'Children don't do what you **tell** them, they do what you **do**'.

This might be more easily understood as children learn by **watching** others and mirroring or mimicking them (words and actions) rather than by **listening to the verbal instructions** of others. Therefore be **careful** what you do because **what you do, - you teach!**

The biggest problem by far in terms of dental disease is the overuse and wrong use of sugar. This is a problem with Western society in general. We are doing a number of things in relation to this, which do not serve us well.

First of all we have a tendency to use sugar as comfort.

Indeed this is true of food in general but particularly sugar. When children are upset, parents or guardians often give something sweet to 'cheer them up'. Another example is an old practice of dipping an infant's dummy into sugar to stop them crying. This is known to produce what is described as 'rampant decay' in the baby teeth where the entire set, upper and lower, are devastated by tooth decay. Thankfully that practice is no longer common although we still see it from time to time.

The point is that it is wise to resist using sugar as comfort for our children.

When the child is crying simply stay with it and hold it, cuddle it and soothe it with your voice, talking or humming or singing gently to it. I can easily appreciate that the parents may be worried or anxious themselves and can easily get panicky if a child is crying. You often hear people saying that they would 'try anything to shut them up'. This is not a good policy and tends to aggravate the situation rather than help.

It is also wise to resist using sugar as a reward.

Very often parents use sugar (sweet) as a reward for getting children to do things or to behave well. 'If you do this or that I will get you something nice'. This is not a helpful practice. Once again it leads to associations in the child's mind. This pattern, if established, can lead to a kind of dependence on sugar. When things are not going according to plan or where things have to be done that you would prefer not to do, there is the tendency to 'sweeten' yourself with sweet things. This becomes a kind of stress behaviour pattern and continues into adult life. It could be considered as a 'sugar addiction'.

It is also important that sugar (sweet things) should not be forbidden to the child.

Many people, on learning that sugar frequency is a major factor in tooth decay, decide that sugar should be banned. This is not a good policy for a number of reasons.

Firstly, sugar (carbohydrate) is one of three basic food-types and to ban it is to ban at least one third of foods available. This is clearly **extremely limiting** in terms of what a child can eat in that a great number of foodstuffs contain sugar.

Secondly, every child deserves a treat. Banning sugar outright can cause the child to feel cheated. This can either cause outright revolt or even worse, the child will hide feelings of resentment which could fester inside over time as they watch friends and other children being allowed what is denied to them. This could be a source of great unhappiness for the child, as anyone could easily imagine.

Thirdly, it is foolish to invest responsibility in the foodstuff instead of the people using it!

Remember that it is **how you use the food** and not the food itself.

It is always best to avoid extremes (all or nothing) and walk the path of balance.

Establish good eating routines with the children, discouraging frequent snacking. If frequent snacking is a problem, there is a strong likelihood the child is using food as a comfort and probably needs some emotional support and maybe even counselling. Gentleness is so important in these instances in discovering if they are worried about something at home or at school perhaps. Let them know that you are on their side and take whatever action may be necessary to reassure them that the problem can be solved.

Make space for their emotions

Children need space for their emotions. It is especially important that they can express frustration and anger safely without risking the disapproval of the parent. Where there is no space for a child's emotions (feelings), and in particular the child's negative feelings, many undesirable consequences follow. Firstly, if there is no safe space to express (or allow out), these negative feelings must remain inside. The result, even in children, is stress. As these feelings get buried on a regular basis, it becomes habitual. Ultimately, suppression (stuffing down) becomes the unconscious reaction to all unwanted (negative) feeling/emotion. This can set the stage for a lifetime of struggle with negative emotion (stress) and indeed is the very reason why our need for stress management is so acute in these times.

This is why ensuring a safe and loving place to express feelings is the greatest gift a parent can give a child. It allows the child to build a sense of comfort, understanding and security even in the difficult times. It also cultivates the same qualities in the child for other people. What price can we put on such a gift?

Encourage plenty of physical playing and exercise.

Plenty of physical playing and exercise encourages a healthy hunger for meals and is necessary for good health and development. Remember that 'hunger is good sauce' and use this to promote good eating habits.

It is the parent's role to act as wise authors and guardians of the daily menu.

I am sure that many of you have noticed that we as parents are tending to lose our stewardship of the diet in the household. With the very best intention of giving choice to the children, we ask them what they want. Children cannot distinguish between what they want and what they need and so given the choice they will be very inclined to choose only sweet taste. It is so important that parents retake the guardian's role in relation to diet.

When children get used to determining diet, it is not an easy task to restore parental guidance. Therefore it is preferable to begin as you mean to continue but it is never too late to change. Sadly this loss of parental stewardship is very common throughout society and leads to so much anguish and strife in the home.

Being too forceful and demanding and allowing no choice is an **equally** poor strategy. **The path of balance is always the better option.** Allow them a choice between two or three items rather than the choice of 'What do you want?'

It is well for us as parents to remember the old adage "practice what you preach".

This can be the hard bit. It behoves us as parents to take a very careful and honest look at ourselves. How can we ask children to do something that we are not prepared to do ourselves? It is almost guaranteed that if children are displaying an over-fondness for sweet things, one or both of the parents will have that same behaviour or habit. Addressing the problem in ourselves **first** as **adults** will achieve more easily the results we desire.

Example is the best teacher.

Cultivating good eating habits is best done by **sharing those habits** with your children. Food is a delight to be enjoyed, - literally to be a source of joy. Unfortunately, society has cultivated many unhelpful notions around food.

The idea that it is something you have to do to stay alive is often overemphasized. When that happens, food can become a chore forced on the children and the dinner table can become a daily battlefield. This can become very distressing for the child as well as for the parent. Parents can be very forceful in their methods from a pressurized cajoling to angry insisting and right up to aggression and smacking. It is not difficult to see how emotional/psychological issues can be easily created around food, so taking away any possible enjoyment.

Society has also created a fashion around food in advertising, especially on television. It seems that there is an emphasis on creating 'needs' in people for the purpose of profit. It is well that people be aware of how easily manipulation and exploitation can occur in circumstances like these. I wonder how often are possible negative consequences to the individual considered when advertising and marketing strategies are devised. It is as well to be aware of this when choosing products to buy.

So be aware and choose with care.

You may have noticed that we have hardly mentioned teeth at all.

This is because, in truth, there is usually little wrong with the teeth themselves. The problem is in how our behaviours can affect the health of the teeth. This means that if we change attitudes and behaviours we will have little in the way of dental disease.

This may sound surprising at first. But it is no different from saying that the problem of nail biting, which destroys the nails, has nothing very much to do with the nails. It is the behaviour of biting them, which destroys them. Change the behaviour and the problem is solved without touching the nails.

So it is with the teeth, change the behaviours and the dental problems are solved.

Summary Of Advice To Parents

- Always begin with yourself

- Make sure that you do what you expect your children to do

- Cultivate good eating habits, - food for nutrition and enjoyment

- Teach them to always express how they feel, - make it safe for them to speak their minds

- Make sure they have their treats, - but not for comfort, reward or emotional support

- Avoid using food as comfort or reward

- Avoid using food as emotional support

- Avoid blaming the food, - change the behaviour instead

- Avoid the pattern of frequent snacking

- Cultivate playing and physical exercise to produce a healthy hunger

- Maintain parental stewardship of the daily menu

- Choose quality foods and products

- Be aware of the seduction of big company food advertising

The preservation of a child's native esteem is far more important than the acquisition of technical skills.

~ Ken Carey

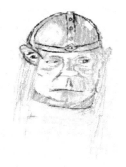

Chapter 14

The Mouth Is The Mirror Of The Body

Chapter 14.

The Mouth is the Mirror of the Body

Clean but the mirror, and the message that shines forth from what the mirror holds out for everyone to see, no one can fail to understand.
~A Course in Miracles

We have seen now the origins of common dental disease. We have made our journey from mind to body using the gentle light of understanding as our guide. We begin to realise that the patterns in the mouth are reflections of our ideas and notions about ourselves. These ideas and notions are reflected through the mirror of the feelings and emotions. Those feelings and emotions reflect in our behaviours and habits and in the same way, the habits and behaviours reflect the condition of the mouth and teeth.

Your Mouth Speaks To You

The reflections do not stop there. The same habits and behaviours that show themselves in the mouth also affect the body in general. For example, if a person has a problem with comfort eating, that person will have difficulty with weight management. Such a person will tend to be overweight. We know that being overweight increases the risk of heart disease and the tendency to increased blood pressure. It may also pose problems with cholesterol and arterial disease. Diabetes is also a greater risk with the tendency to be overweight. This relates to the same pattern as tooth decay with a person tending to be "addicted" to sweet things.

The pattern of disease in a person's mouth is therefore indicating general patterns in a person's health and life. A map of the disease patterns in the mouth is a map of **general patterns of disease** in the body. In understanding this, you can use the information and insight gleaned from your dental patterns and trends, to point the way to your general health and well-being. In this way your mouth speaks to you, pointing out the issues which need to be addressed in order to bring to you the excellent health which is yours to enjoy. As such then, the mouth is the mirror of the body. The issues pointed out in the mouth will mirror the general issues, which can then be addressed, and so move you toward health. To begin to understand the mouth as the mirror of the body, let us examine the various aspects of the functions of the mouth and how they impact the body in a general way.

Your Mouth is The Gateway of Your Body.

Consider that almost all that is given entry to the body is given entry through the mouth. The main item here is food, but we can also include the smoking of tobacco and other substances and the drinking of alcohol. Let's begin with food, the basic sustenance of the body. This represents the **Mouth as the Organ of Nourishment**

and Sustenance. Let us look at the consequences of a problem relationship with food.

Our relationship with food has many and varied consequences for our health. The first and most obvious is management of weight. However, other conditions such as health of heart and health of arteries, as well as health of pancreas and health of bowels, are all directly related to our relationship with food.

Notice all the organs that we have mentioned in the same breath as food. We first mentioned weight and we know that blood pressure and heart problems are related to weight problems. Disease of the arteries (cholesterol) is also related to the food we consume. Blood pressure in turn affects the kidneys and the bladder. Problems with the stomach are also associated with eating. Our relationship with sweet taste has consequences for our teeth but also for the pancreas and this, of course, has consequences in terms of insulin and diabetes.

Is it not interesting that almost all of our worst problems with disease in society have been mentioned in the same breath as food? Even diseases such as cancer have been linked with various aspects of our diet. This is such an important statement.

Beware, however, not to make the mistake of blaming the food. It is we who decide what substances are placed in the mouth. It is we who decide what we eat and drink. Therefore we must be responsible for the consequences of our decisions and our actions.

If we look at other substances to which we allow entry, e.g. cigarette smoke and alcohol, we find an association with many more of our problematic diseases. Cigarettes (cigars etc.) we associate with sore mouth, gum disease and sore throat as well as bronchitis and lung diseases and even mouth and lung cancer. Alcohol we associate with diseases of the liver, among others. Already we have mentioned most if not all of society's worst plagues. It follows that if we correct our relationship with food and other substances all these organs must benefit and improve their health accordingly.

Don't beat yourself up!

This is in no way intended to make a person feel bad **because** they smoke or drink, or because they have a weight problem, or because they have the habit of clenching and grinding or because they have **any** habit or condition. Indeed I would ask that people understand that it is **because** they feel bad that they smoke or drink or harbour any habit. So feeling bad about feeling bad is definitely **not** the way to go!

I urge you to be gentle with yourself. Don't expect too much too soon. Steady progress is the way to go!

It's a Two Way Gateway

As well as giving entry through the mouth, we also use the mouth as an exit. It is the gateway through which we express ourselves. We speak, we laugh, we cry, we shout, we sing. We express ourselves, our thoughts and feelings. It is our channel of communication. We recognise the

Mouth as the Organ of Communication and consider the relationship that we have with speaking our minds, expressing our feelings. This particular relationship has implications for our psychological and emotional health as well as the health of the jaws, teeth and gums.

When we 'keep the mouth shut' for whatever reason we deny this function of the mouth. Our feelings are denied expression and we 'bottle it up'. Although the consequences of this are most obviously emotional and psychological, the stress that results will tend to promote the seeking of comfort in eating, eating sweet things, smoking or drinking or other habits. The psychological and emotional stress also manifests physically in the habit of clenching and grinding the teeth and this has direct physical consequences for the tissues in the mouth as we have seen. This brings us back complete circle to the problem relationship with food and other substances. It is clear then that both problems are intimately related. Indeed they are inseparable from each other and inseparable from the vicious cycle that they engender.

We also respect the **Mouth as the Organ of Enjoyment and Pleasure,** allowing us to experience an infinite range of flavours, textures and tastes. This relationship has implications for psychological and emotional health as well, in that enjoyment and pleasure is sometimes seen in some cultures as wrong, selfish or 'sinful'. This notion of sinfulness is often particularly associated with sexual pleasure and enjoyment and the mouth plays a major role in kissing and sexual intimacy. These notions are commonplace in Irish society and in many other societies and engender intense levels and quantities of shame and guilt around sexual matters. The emotions of shame and guilt are very powerful stressors and play an enormous role in preventing emotional and psychological well-being in the individual. This area alone needs a lot of understanding and education but that is quite another day's work and not within the scope of this book.

Your Wealth Is Your Health

Excellent health is within your easy reach. It is not a pipe dream, impossible to realise, but an achievable goal for everyone. It will **not** be bought with **money**, no matter how big is the bank account. It will **not** be achieved through taking pills and medicines, although pills and medicines may be an enormous help to you along the way. It will **not** be achieved through undergoing procedures and operations, although these procedures and operations may also be necessary in certain situations.

It is achieved through the commitment to understand the nature of negative thought patterns and the resultant stress (negative emotional patterns) that they create. It is achieved by recognising that these habits and behaviours are supported by the stress matrix. It is achieved as we offer the willingness to make adjustments in life-style to dissolve stress and support new health-promoting habits and behaviours.

The gains in health that the tissues of the mouth enjoy are mirrored in every tissue, as we move forward, step by step, towards perfect health. All components are addressed, mind, emotion and body. No part is ignored or left untreated.

Healthy Body ~ Healthy Mind

We have all heard these "old sayings" but few have understood the profound wisdom in them. Maybe we would be better to say instead "Healthy Mind ~ Healthy Body" since mind is always the starting point, but the old wisdom of putting them side by side seems to have been forgotten in modern healthcare. This forgetting has cost us very dearly indeed, not just in terms of enormous amounts of money, but much more seriously, in terms of the enormous amounts of pain and suffering we have generated and continue to generate for ourselves. Understanding mind as origin, and emotion (feeling) as the vehicle carrying and supporting habits and behaviours, is the key to bringing about the changes in habits and behaviours, which will produce in the body the health that we all desire.

All phenomena are mind, mind is all. Mind contains rivers, mountains, moon and sun.

~ Japenese Zen master, Dogen.

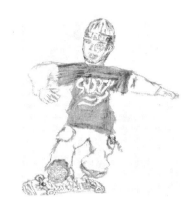

Chapter 15

What's It All About, Anyway?

Chapter 15.

What's It All About, Anyway?

The problems that exist in the world cannot be solved by the level of thinking that created them.
~ Albert Einstein.

Negative human behaviour/habit is the source of societies' greatest ills. Consider drug addiction for a moment. Remember that addictions are simply more extreme habits where the substance used is seen as a life and death issue. A person genuinely believes that they cannot live without it! Their negative thought patterns and the stress that is produced by them are severe and extreme. **This stress is often an all-consuming terror of life without the substance.**

Heroin and other "heavy drug" addictions have inflicted and continue to inflict the most horrific suffering on our society. Alcoholism, the more acceptable first cousin, is also wreaking havoc in families and communities. The pain and suffering caused is emotional and psychological as well as physical and involves so many more people than just the addicts themselves. Indeed all are affected, from the individual, through the family, to the community and society in general. Smoking, the even more acceptable addiction in society, is related to much physical illness and tremendously expensive treatment. Indeed expensive treatment is common to all addictions and the effects of addictions, but **never guaranteed** to work. Maybe the reason that our treatments are so singularly unsuccessful has become clearer as we finish our journey of understanding through the human side of dental disease. After all dental disease is just disease in a specific system (the mouth) and thus shares the common attributes of all disease in other systems.

In a sentence, we are attempting to treat an effect (the end product) without reference to the cause (the source or origin). What hope of success could come from this?

This is very simply why so many common strategies fail so many people. More and more money is spent on healthcare for less and less in terms of results. Everybody has someone else to blame for the failure of the healthcare system, missing the essential point that the **system itself** is inherently flawed. No amount of reform, however expensive or radical, can bring success to a machine with such major design faults that it can never fulfill its function. The machine needs to be redesigned, not repaired.

How has science failed us?

The answer is again simple. Science is a pursuit of our human species, yet it neglects anything that it cannot measure. But many of the fundamental characteristics of humanity cannot **be** measured. This is especially true of emotions. Science then chooses to ignore a major facet of human life, - our emotional life. This facet of human life is so woven into the very fabric of our daily existence, both work and leisure, that to ignore it is to omit a vital ingredient of our humanity. Science then fails humanity because it does not honour all of our humanness. It cannot speak to the whole when it operates only in part.

It has long been recognized that knowledge alone is not enough to change behaviour. Knowing the dangers of smoking does not stop intelligent people from smoking. Knowing the possible fatal consequences of drug addiction does not prevent intelligent and highly creative people from falling prey. Why do so many of us, including highly acclaimed stars of music, screen and sports, fall prey to drugs? What is it about us as a people that makes us even more likely to fall prey, when we have fame and fortune?

The answer lies in our poor understanding of stress, - our negative feelings and emotions, - and how these form the **supporting matrix** for our habits and behaviours. We also do not appreciate how these habits and behaviours support the disease process physically. That is why it is crucial for us as individuals and as community to begin the integration of our various fields of study to see how they are related and interrelated. No field of health science is complete without the relevant psychology and behavioural science. This is how we honour **wisdom** rather than **knowledge** and find the way to change the behaviours that do not serve us or our good health.

Changing behaviours - what does not work!

The traditional **methods** for **behavioural change** do <u>**not**</u> work. Once again the problem is that we put the focus on the habit /behaviour. We seek to "stamp it out". We will force change. We will punish negative behaviour. Those engaged in negative behaviour will be singled out, pressurized, condemned, fined, or jailed.

These methods do not work because they increase the stress levels in the individuals concerned. The supporting matrix (stress, negative emotion) for habits and behaviours is actually increased and fortified by this type of intervention. This means that the habits, far from being undone, are actually increased and strengthened by the very effort to remove them. The greater the effort put into this type of intervention the worse the problem becomes. This is the reason that we need more and more jail spaces to house an increasing number of offenders. It is also the reason that the level of alcohol abuse is increasing among young people, as is the addiction to smoking increasing among young people. This is all the proof that one needs to show that the methods we employ are not only ineffective but are actually counterproductive.

Changing behaviours - what *can* work!

The way to change behaviours and habits is to understand how they originate and the matrix of negative emotions and feelings (stress) that supports them. When we begin to tackle this stress matrix we will begin to see results. Dismantling the stress matrix is not an easy task. For the individual, family and community it requires care, commitment, patience and time.

Stress management in its various guises can be introduced into the school curriculum for teachers and for pupils. Parents too, should be given the opportunity to benefit from this practice. Counselling should be available easily to everyone, young and old, as **primary care**. This would allow people to learn how to deal with dangerous negative emotions in a controlled and caring environment.

People should never be put under pressure to break a habit, either by condemnation, penalty or fine. People who choose to continue with habits cannot and should not be forced to comply. Hopefully, in time, the negative outcomes produced by the habits will cause them to want to choose another path. This type of policy may seem to condone the negative behaviour and might be viewed as supporting it. This is not the case.

Trying to force the behaviour to stop is what will actually support it!

This cannot be repeated often enough. It needs to be clearly understood as a fundamental principle. So much time and genuine good will, as well as money and other precious resources, are wasted on useless and outmoded methods. Now is the time to begin putting our resources into methods that will actually produce results.

Physician heal thyself

Your best resource for health is yourself. Taking time (and courses) to understand more about the human condition in its wholeness, - body, mind and spirit will provide you with invaluable tools and information to begin to take charge of your own health and well-being. Help is always available from your health-care professionals as you journey on your way. There is no hurry and no rush. Every effort brings you closer to your goal.

I wish you every blessing on your journey.

If there is any primary rule of science, it is...acceptance of the obligation to acknowledge and describe all of reality, all that exists, everything that is the case...It must accept within its jurisdiction even that which it cannot understand, explain, that for which no theory exists, that which cannot be measured, predicted, controlled or ordered...It includes all levels or stages of knowledge, including the inchoate...knowledge of low reliability,...and subjective experience.

~ *Abraham Maslow*

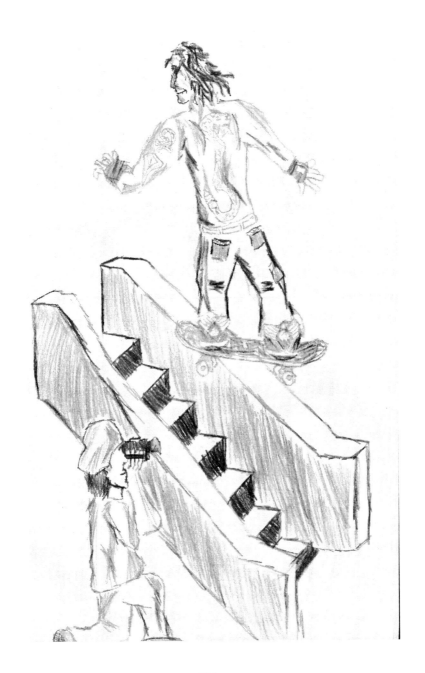

People As Partners in Medicine

People as Partners in Medicine is an organisation dedicated to **people power** in the promotion of Health, the care of Health, and the prevention of disease. The principles that are outlined in **"Something To Chew On"** form the basis of the 'People As Partners' approach. We recognize and welcome the **Whole Person, - Mind, Emotion, Body and Spirit.**

We aim to support people in their caring for their own health and wellbeing. We aim to bring the latest in education and understanding to the field of healthcare and to **raise people to the position of partner with the doctor/therapist.**

One the one hand, people recognise the limitations of modern medicine as well as its great benefits. On the other, people begin to recognize that their greatest resource is themselves. As they do, the door to this treasure trove swings open and the jewels of wisdom and understanding are claimed as natural inheritance. Power is re-sourced, - sourced again, not from without this time, but from within.

Excellent health for everybody is not just a pipe dream, but a realistic and achievable goal pursued on a daily basis. At present, many people give nothing to their health on a daily basis, often asking too much of the body and giving only the bare minimum in return. When, after many years, health begins to fail or we end up with a health crisis, we suddenly realise how valuable a gift is good health and regret the lost opportunity.

Is it not in your own best interest to begin Daily Health Care?

Learn to enhance the health of your mind.

Learn to enhance your emotional health.

Learn to enhance your physical health.

Learn to enhance your spiritual health.

Become a joyful, happy and fulfilled person getting the maximum out of your work and your life. That is our vision for everyone. Our heartfelt desire is to help you achieve it.

        People As Partners can be reached at
        www.peopleaspartnersinmedicine.com

ISBN 141201381-X